Rehabilitation for Traumatic Brain Injury

For Churchill Livingstone:

Editorial Director: Mary Law
Project Manager: Gail Murray
Project Development Manager: Dinah Thom
Designer: George Ajayi

Rehabilitation for Traumatic Brain Injury
Physical Therapy Practice in Context

Maggie Campbell MCSP SRP
Research Physiotherapist, NHS Trent; formerly Lead Clinician Physiotherapist, Head Injury Rehabilitation Centre, Sheffield, UK

Foreword by

Andy Tyerman BA MSc PhD CPsychol
Consultant Clinical Psychologist, Community Head Injury Service, Bedgrove Health Centre, Aylesbury, UK

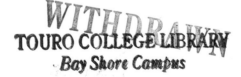

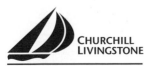

CHURCHILL
LIVINGSTONE

EDINBURGH LONDON NEW YORK PHILADELPHIA ST LOUIS SYDNEY TORONTO 2000

MT-HS

CHURCHILL LIVINGSTONE
An imprint of Harcourt Publishers Limited

© Harcourt Publishers Limited 2000

⟁ is a registered trademark of Harcourt Publishers Limited

First published 2000

ISBN 0 443 06131 9

British Library Cataloguing in Publication Data
A catalogue record for this book is available from the British Library

Library of Congress Cataloging in Publication Data
A catalog record for this book is available from the Library of Congress

Note
Medical knowledge is constantly changing. As new information becomes available, changes in treatment, procedures, equipment and the use of drugs become necessary. The author and the publishers have, as far as it is possible, taken care to ensure that the information given in this text is accurate and up to date. However, readers are strongly advised to confirm that the information, especially with regard to drug usage, complies with the latest legislation and standards of practice.

The
publisher's
policy is to use
**paper manufactured
from sustainable forests**

Printed in China

11/25/02

Contents

Foreword

Rehabilitation after traumatic brain injury (TBI) is immensely complex and challenging with so much for even the experienced professional still to learn This book makes a valuable contribution to both clinical practice and service planning. This is achieved through thoughtful analysis of philosophical, theoretical and clinical issues drawing on the author's obvious wealth of clinical experience, supported by key summaries, case examples and practical suggestions. While obviously of particular interest to those involved in physical therapy, the book would in my view be an informative and constructive read for all members of the rehabilitation team.

You may wonder what a clinical neuropsychologist, albeit one with specialist expertise in rehabilitation after traumatic brain injury, is doing writing the foreword to a book about physical therapy – so, initially, did I. My reaction when first approached was one of surprise and some concern – what do I know about physiotherapy? The key to my involvement lies in the subtitle 'Physical therapy practice *in context*'. When it was explained that the book sought to place physical therapy in the context of the rehabilitation team, I was reassured that it was appropriate for me to write the foreword. As we have developed our Community Head Injury Service in Aylesbury, I have always viewed the Head Injury Rehabilitation Centre in Sheffield as being one of our closest parallels in both service provision and philosophy.

I anticipated a book which provided an account of physiotherapy after TBI in the context of inter- or trans-disciplinary team working. On reading the book the context for physical therapy is much broader and deeper. A client-centred and holistic approach is advocated, anchoring both assessment and rehabilitation firmly in the life context of both the person with TBI and their family. It is suggested that the benefits of such an approach lie both in contributing to the setting of appropriate and meaningful goals and in reducing the potential for conflict, thereby maximizing our collective efforts to achieve progress in rehabilitation. By adopting such an approach in advance of goal planning or direct intervention, is it is asserted that workload is lessened rather than increased. In my experience, anchoring our interventions in an understanding of the personal and family context increases greatly the chances of positive engagement on the part of the client and of establishing an effective working partnership with the family. It also provides the foundation for promoting positive long-term adaptation for both the client and family. While many of us would endorse the need to negotiate goals with clients and families, this is a highly skilled task after TBI, one that is rarely addressed in professional training programmes.

The process of inter-disciplinary assessment, the foundation for effective rehabilitation, is addressed in depth. The process of 'global' and 'holistic' assessment is detailed, along with an assessment template. While, as a clinical neuropsychologist, I am not qualified to comment on sensorimotor assessment, this section provided me with a valuable insight into the rationale for and practice of physiotherapy assessment.

This is followed by an account of a carefully crafted inter-disciplinary assessment case discussion and goal setting process, illustrated by detailed case examples. This is likely to prove instructive for professionals inexperienced in TBI rehabilitation or new to the complexities of interdisciplinary teamwork, as well as those seeking to improve the functioning of their own brain injury rehabilitation team.

I found the account of neurophysiotherapy to be fascinating. I was surprised to learn that clinical practice had developed independently from its scientific knowledge base, having previously assumed that physical treatments had a strong theoretical as well as empirical base. I was intrigued to learn that training has tended to emphasize technique rather than its evidential base, especially coming from a profession which stresses the 'scientist–practitioner model', sometimes, in my view, at the expense of core clinical skills.

After a critique of the current state of neurophysiotherapy, current clinical practice in TBI is reviewed with illustrative examples. It is concluded that there is 'much to do to develop practice based on best evidence', with a particular need for research and evaluation specific to TBI. The author makes a plea for all practitioners to contribute to further development of the knowledge base, either by direct research or through engaging in evaluative discussion. An integrated approach involving cross-validation of experiential and experimentally derived knowledge is advocated.

One of the most valuable features of this book is the discussion of how cognitive and behavioural difficulties impact on physiotherapy. Common behavioural difficulties and the need to understand underlying cognitive limitations in the assessment process are discussed along with an illustrative case example. This is followed by excellent practical suggestions about the management of such difficulties, again illustrated with a case example. Specific suggestions are provided for the management of difficulties with adjustment, attention, inappropriate behaviour and fatigue. It is argued that with guidance from the team the physiotherapist can not only reduce restrictions imposed by cognitive and behavioural difficulties within physiotherapy, but also promote clients' engagement in other aspects of the rehabilitation programme and contribute to social skills, behavioural, communication and cognitive rehabilitation programmes. The inter-dependent nature of rehabilitation and the need for effective team-working is rightfully stressed but of course this is not easily achieved. The head injury rehabilitation team in Sheffield clearly worked hard to achieve an impressive degree of clinical integration.

Finally, rehabilitation after TBI is placed in the context of the wider healthcare system. The comments about the difficulty in developing good practice in the context of rapid organizational change will resonate among rehabilitation professionals within the NHS. The need for a higher profile for rehabilitation with greater representation in healthcare planning will be endorsed throughout the TBI community. The book concludes with recommendations about the provision of rehabilitation services. Professionals working in TBI need to strive for greater recognition of the value of rehabilitation and wider representation in healthcare planning if such recommendations are to be realized.

In conclusion, there is much to commend in this book in its contribution not only to the provision of physiotherapy services but also in highlighting the benefits of a client-centred, holistic approach to rehabilitation after TBI. The author lays down an explicit challenge to neurophysiotherapists to develop their knowledge base and to play a full role in the rehabilitation process. There is also an implicit challenge to all rehabilitation professionals, especially to neurophysiotherapists and neuropsychologists, to pool our knowledge and work more closely in the context of the inter-disciplinary team in order to optimize the benefits of our interventions for clients with TBI and their families.

Andy Tyerman

Preface

Single pathology texts aimed primarily at physiotherapists are still relatively rare. However, the complex nature of traumatic brain injury (TBI) means that it can be covered only superficially within multi-pathology texts. This book focuses solely on TBI to help the reader develop a deeper understanding of the pathology and effects of any significant traumatic insult to the brain. While the subject matter of the text is focused, I believe that many of the issues covered, and the suggestions offered, relate directly to other areas of neurorehabilitation. Equally, although the text has been developed for physiotherapists, much of the content may prove useful to other members of the rehabilitation team and to other professionals involved in the planning, management or evaluation of TBI services. I hope that this book is accessible enough to provide a basic text for undergraduate therapists as well as meeting the needs of practising therapists looking to extend their knowledge, deepen their understanding, or find specific guidance. I hope also that the ideas presented will promote discussion within the physiotherapy profession and result in increased levels of regular practice evaluation and a flurry of research activity! Most of all, I hope that this book will in some way help to improve the management of individuals who sustain a traumatic brain injury.

This book results from a lengthy process of personal and professional development that has been prompted and sustained with the assistance of very many individuals. It would be impossible to acknowledge everyone who has made a contribution and therefore the following represents just the edited highlights.

I would like to thank Margaret Reid for teaching me the value of observational skills, and John Reid, who first made me aware of the value of organized teamwork when striving for a common goal. I acknowledge the influence of the staff of the Institute of Neurological Sciences, Glasgow, whose passion and professionalism first stimulated my interest in TBI and who provided me with a sound cross-disciplinary education in all things neuro between 1979 and 1984.

My working life at the Head Injury Rehabilitation Centre (HIRC), Sheffield, has been the most challenging and the most rewarding period of my clinical practice. It is difficult to acknowledge the contribution to my professional development made by those who have survived traumatic brain injury, and that made by their friends and families, without sounding trite. However, for me that contribution has been and continues to be vital, providing motivation, inspiration and increased understanding. All HIRC staff have contributed to my learning and I have derived support from many individuals. I would like, therefore, to give special thanks to all of those involved in the development and delivery of the HIRC service from 1988 onwards and to acknowledge their contribution to many of the ideas presented in this book. A better team I have yet to meet.

In part, it seems inappropriate to single out individuals from what has been so much a team process; however, there are a few individuals whose influence I would particularly like to acknowledge. The late Peter Clarke, who gave me permission to comment on psychological issues, Jenny Garber, who helped me to listen better to carers and who provided a seemingly endless supply of innovative commonsense solutions; Richard Body, who helped me understand the value for all in defining limits of responsibility and who has improved my written work just a little; Carole Downie, who brought the unruly team members into line so that collaborative note-keeping could become a reality; and Camilla Herbert and Mark Parker, who could always be relied upon to raise the level of discussion. Finally, there are two individuals whose cooperation has been essential to the production of this book. My thanks, therefore, go once more to Richard Body for his support throughout this project and in particular for ploughing through the first draft of every chapter, and a very special mention goes to Patrick Body, who has learned to be possibly the most invisible seven-year-old in the world. Thank you both for your patience.

Sheffield 2000   Maggie Campbell

Abbreviations

ADL	Activities of daily living	**NHIF**	National Head Injury Foundation
CNS	Central nervous system		
CPP	Cerebral perfusion pressure	**NHS**	National Health Service
		NIH	National Institutes of Health
CSF	Cerebrospinal fluid		
CT	Computed tomography	**PET**	Positron emission tomography
DAI	Diffuse axonal injury		
EEG	Electroencephalography	**PNF**	Proprioceptive neuromuscular facilitation
EMG	Electromyography		
fMRI	Functional magnetic resonance imaging	**PPC**	Posterior parietal cortex
GCS	Glasgow Coma Scale/Score	**PTA**	Post-traumatic amnesia
		PVS	Persistent vegetative state
GOAT	Galveston orientation and amnesia test		
		ROM	Range of movement
GP	General practitioner	**TBI**	Traumatic brain injury
HO	Heterotopic ossification	**TMS**	Transcranial magnetic stimulation
ICP	Intracranial pressure		
ICU	Intensive care unit	**VOR**	Vestibulo-ocular reflex
MABP	Mean arterial blood pressure	**WHIM**	Wessex Head Injury Matrix

1

About this book

Key Points

- A client-centred approach is necessary for reasons of effectiveness and efficiency
- Physiotherapists need to access direct support from, and the published literature of, other disciplines
- The role of physiotherapists in TBI rehabilitation beyond acute care has yet to be adequately defined or its development supported by systematic programmes of postgraduate education
- Physiotherapists have significant potential to increase their contribution to TBI rehabilitation; this book presents a conceptual framework designed to facilitate such an aim

THE PHILOSOPHY OF THIS BOOK

This book describes an approach to traumatic brain injury (TBI) rehabilitation that attempts to place the individual who has sustained the injury, their family and their friends at the centre of the process. This approach, by placing emphasis on the needs of individuals requiring a service, demands that the professionals providing that service look outward towards the real world and to real lives; to see the wider landscape from which their clients come and back into which they would reasonably hope to return. It is an attempt to outline in practical terms how the skills and knowledge of individual physiotherapists, and those of the wider physiotherapeutic profession, can be harnessed in the most efficient and effective way to address some of the most challenging issues in rehabilitation practice.

This practical process is based around identifying a wide range of potential influences on the individual who has sustained the injury and then considering the impact of those influences on the physiotherapeutic assessment process as an integral part of that assessment and *in advance of embarking on any programme of intervention*. This contrasts with a still common approach where physical deficits are assessed, and physical goals set, often in isolation from other rehabilitation goals and sometimes without sufficient consideration of the potential functional outcome.

There are many positive results of taking a more considered approach. These include the development of an appropriate level of expectation of the immediate outcome of the present intervention, the recognition of when intervention is not appropriate and, when placed in the context of interdisciplinary team intervention, an increased chance of achieving an outcome for individuals that is meaningful in terms of their lifestyle.

Thus, within this philosophical approach, physiotherapists who work with someone who has sustained a TBI are encouraged to understand the context within which they are providing a specialist assessment of physical status and physiotherapeutic needs, and in understanding that context, to develop holistic practice in terms of assessment, intervention and longer-term management.

POTENTIATING THERAPEUTIC OUTCOMES

In describing the physiotherapist's role in this way, the suggestion is not that the physiotherapist should embark on hours of assessment of, for example, cognitive ability, nor is it suggested that the physiotherapist should become skilled in family therapy. It is anticipated, however, that the physiotherapist will recognize the importance of knowing what cognitive restrictions an individual has when planning and delivering an intervention. Similarly, it should be understood that a client's previous life and their present circumstances will have a strong influence on the ultimate outcome of any rehabilitation programme.

With a sound knowledge of the individual's strengths and limitations, the physiotherapist is able to plan appropriately the content, pace and progression of direct sessions, and to anticipate a realistic level of self-direction from the injured person. With a clear understanding of the level of support available to that person and also of the demands being made by family, friends and other rehabilitation professionals, the physiotherapist can design a home programme that is feasible and appropriate to the individual's circumstances. Knowledge of the wider context allows the physiotherapist to anticipate barriers to progress and predict the final outcome more realistically.

This book, then, promotes the idea of setting realistic goals based on knowledge and gathering adequate knowledge in order to set realistic goals. Neurophysiotherapists possess a great deal of knowledge concerning the assessment of sensorimotor dysfunction. They are skilled observers of how dysfunctional movement relates to the range of normal functional movement. They are proficient in methods of facilitating more normal sensorimotor experiences for those with dysfunction and in aiding them to relearn efficient and effective motor action. They assist many individuals to progress positively along the abnormal–normal movement continuum and prevent others from regressing. However, many practitioners recognize that there are individuals who do not progress in the way that would be expected or hoped for.

Often, treatment failures are explained in terms of the injured individual's lack of application, their lack of motivation or apparent lack of effort. While it is accepted that there will always be individuals whom professionals will fail to reach, there are others whose apparent disinterest can be explained by coexisting difficulties such as poor planning skills or low levels of arousal. In some cases, environmental factors such as cultural influences or social and family role demands may be limiting factors.

The approach outlined in this book suggests that by adopting a more proactive approach to the gathering and sharing of information, by adopting a more holistic approach to their practice, neurophysiotherapists can achieve better outcomes for a wider range of people with whom they work. It is also anticipated that inexperienced therapists and those who have specialized in other areas of physiotherapy practice will find this a useful reference book and guide when their practice brings them into contact with someone who has in the past sustained a TBI.

DEFINING AN APPROACH TO INTERVENTION

Holistic practice is an ideal that is far from easy to achieve. This book is not a text of absolute answers but it does attempt to frame a number of the questions to help identify some of the answers. It also advances some basic assessment and intervention ideas and some specific opinions. Rehabilitation following TBI is a young discipline, and physiotherapeutic practice within this discipline is equally young. Thus, many of our interventions, and those of our colleagues in other rehabilitation professions, are not described within the literature. Documentation of the outcome of specific interventions is limited and evidence of the efficacy of intervention beyond the acute stage is particularly scarce (Watson 1997).

Building on clinical experience

However, in recognizing the paucity of published evidence, the accumulation of successful clinical experience should not be ignored, particularly where success is represented by functionally valid outcomes. Much of what is presented in this book in terms of intervention strategies represents practice developed from extensive clinical experience, my own and that of many generous colleagues. In particular it draws on the learning of the last decade, working in a community-based setting, developing an interdisciplinary team in an attempt to meet the complex needs of a wide group of individuals who, having survived a TBI and returned home, often find their lives unrecognizable. As well as the lessons learned from solving problems as each new client has presented them, I have gained much by reading the literature of other disciplines and from discussion with others working in this field. In terms of developing and modifying treatment techniques and approaches, a great deal of my knowledge has come from observing and listening to my clients and those who are close to them.

It is not a new phenomenon for physiotherapeutic practice to be in advance of scientific evidence. When I started my academic and clinical education 20 years ago, stroke rehabilitation was in its infancy. The scientific evidence said simply that a dead dendrite was a dead dendrite and the received wisdom was that people who suffered a cerebrovascular accident with resultant hemiplegia should simply be taught to compensate with the non-affected side. Physiotherapists who argued from clinical experience that better outcomes could be achieved by attempting to restore a level of symmetry and by encouraging relearning of skilled movements were regarded at best as eccentric. However, for those who practised these approaches to treatment, and for those who observed the positive clinical outcomes, there was no doubt that their approach was a valid one.

Support from research findings

Eventually, at least some of the positive clinical observations began to be supported by animal and laboratory studies (e.g. Goldberger & Murray 1980, Greenhough et al 1985), and there is now a wide, although not complete, acceptance of the concept that the neuromuscular system is plastic in healthy and pathological states, i.e. that aspects of the structure and function of the neuromuscular system can change. The implications of the theory of neuromuscular plasticity, that the potential for change can be influenced by extrinsic as well as intrinsic factors, has begun to influence the thinking of many rehabilitation professionals, particularly with reference to the role of repetition and practice. However, there is not as yet a significant body of evidence demonstrating exactly how to harness this plasticity to achieve the most effective intervention.

An approach to therapy

The structure and content of this book, then, is representative of my personal approach to therapy:

- to assess each person as an individual, placing the sensorimotor findings within the context of wider assessment of strengths, limitations, past life and future plans
- to plan interventions using specific evidence where it exists
- to seek out and apply evidence from other disciplines and other areas of practice when available
- to be innovative in the use of clinical reasoning skills when presented with a problem that does not have an obvious solution.

DEVELOPMENTS IN THE MANAGEMENT OF TBI

HISTORICAL PERSPECTIVE

The effects of TBI have long been recognized. In his 1969 text *Patterns of Acute Head Injury*, Hooper (1969) refers to several nineteenth century texts (Abernethy 1811, Guthrie 1847, Macewen 1881) which, in the descriptive style of their time, outline illustrative case studies highlighting the various physical, cognitive and behavioural sequelae of specific types of cranial injuries. However, although they go on to give details of approaches to the medical and surgical management of the life-threatening aspects of the injuries, the rich descriptive detail of the physical and behavioural changes in survivors is not accompanied by any suggestion of intervention.

Like much pathology associated with trauma, an increased understanding of TBI, and some progress in aspects of medical and surgical management, developed over the war years in the first half of the twentieth century. What role, if any, the physiotherapist had within the developing management of the condition remains unclear. However, it is interesting to note that when Cawthorne (1945) and Cooksey (1946) published their work on what we would now refer to as vestibular rehabilitation, they did so in the *Journal of the Chartered Society of Physiotherapy* as well as in the *Proceedings of the Royal Society of Medicine,* and they advocated use of their regime with individuals following TBI.

With technological advances and the escalating demand resultant from the increasing incidence of high-speed road traffic accidents, there were major developments in acute care in the late 1960s and in the 1970s. The focus of medical intervention became clearly based on the prevention of secondary brain damage, and survival rates increased (Jennett & Teasdale 1981). The physiotherapist was by this time identified as a core team member with a particular role in promoting optimal oxygenation of the blood via assessment and maintenance of respiratory function and the physical treatment of respiratory conditions.

DEVELOPING ROLE OF THE PHYSIOTHERAPIST

In parallel to this focus on the prevention of secondary cerebral damage (see Ch. 2) via respiratory care, the physiotherapist also developed a primary role in the prevention of secondary physical changes such as soft tissue contracture and loss of joint range of movement. A model for this combined respiratory and soft tissue maintenance had already been developed in the acute management of poliomyelitis. Thus the most commonly appreciated role of the physiotherapist in the acute management of TBI was established. This role is still recognizable today and continues to form the basis of the physiotherapist's role within the wider team in the acute care of the individual with TBI (Medical Disability Society 1988).

TBI rehabilitation programmes

Over the past two decades physiotherapists have developed a more proactive approach to early management including the development of preventive splinting and have become increasingly involved throughout the inpatient episode, working with other professionals to promote mobility, independence and, hopefully, a return to home and to normality. However, beyond the role in specialist acute care facilities, the extent of physiotherapists' involvement in TBI rehabilitation has evolved inconsistently and has been influenced strongly by the severely limited provision of dedicated TBI rehabilitation services.

In the UK, for example, despite the recognition of the need for specialist services and its repeated documentation in the literature (Burke 1987, Eames & Wood 1989, Hall & Cope 1985, McMillan and Greenwood 1993, McMillan et al 1989), the majority of individuals hospitalized with a TBI continue to be cared for on other specialty wards and often, as in the case of general surgery departments, in an atmosphere of acute illness with no real rehabilitation ethos. Admission policies vary across and within health districts and the number of hospital attenders, the severity of their injuries and the type of associated injuries can fluctuate. Therefore, those individuals admitted with TBI can be allocated a bed in one of a variety of specialisms. Thus, in many settings the critical mass required to highlight needs *locally* has occurred only rarely and specialist posts and rehabilitation teams have been slow to be created. However, in some specialist neurological rehabilitation facilities, for example those established for the treatment of stroke or progressive neurological disorders, teams including physiotherapists have extended their skills to meet the needs of those with TBI (Cockburn and Gatherer 1988). More recently, some facilities previously designated for longer-term care and rehabilitation have accepted the role of providing a more structured approach to inpatient TBI rehabilitation, and many private or charitably funded organizations have set up specific TBI rehabilitation programmes.

The need to extend provision beyond inpatient care has become more readily acknowledged, although dedicated community teams within the UK National Health Service (NHS) are still few in number. Not all post-acute TBI programmes include a physiotherapeutic role and, as many of the scenarios described in the literature are set within a variety of contexts and stem from an almost equally varied range of approaches, the physiotherapeutic role, where it does exist, is not fully consistent across provision.

Service development and education

With these demographic, geographic and philosophical inconsistencies, it has been hard for the physiotherapy profession to be proactive in service development or postgraduate education. This has led to there being an inadequate supply of interested, knowledgeable and skilled physiotherapists available for recruitment particularly at times of increased demand. This was the case when the UK Department of Health enacted a service development initiative in 1992, when funded posts attracted little interest and much of the education in *head injury* had to be provided after employment in a combination of on-the-job experience and attendance at conferences.

At the time of writing, therefore, the physiotherapist is easily seen as part of the acute care team and is always included where an inpatient rehabilitation service is specifically designed to cater for individuals following TBI. As dedicated services are not yet available across wide geographical areas, many physiotherapists with insufficient postgraduate experience continue to encounter people with TBI within their caseload. In line with decreasing length of inpatient stays, these encounters are becoming just as likely for an isolated community therapist as a non-head injury specialist within acute provision. Physiotherapists also encounter individuals many years following injury as they may present at a variety of points of contact with the same range of injuries or conditions as any other member of the public.

DEVELOPMENT OF TBI REHABILITATION

From the content of the previous section it should be understood that the phrase TBI rehabilitation has been used to describe a substantial range of interventions and services, and as such it is virtually impossible to describe a chronological sequence of development.

Elite versus common practice

It is probably fair to say that over the past three decades there have been two parallel developments occurring worldwide. The first might reasonably be described as the development and progression of elite practice and the second as the progression of common practice. Differing professional and economic influences have been at work in different countries throughout this period, leading to specific local developments or barriers to development. In some countries the chasm between elite practice and common practice has been significantly reduced, whereas in others there has been no tangible change in equality of access.

Initial global progress was made in the 1970s with the development and worldwide adoption of the Glasgow Coma Scale (Teasdale & Jennett 1974), which enabled a process of discussion to begin in earnest to try to establish predictors of outcome and comparison of outcomes across different services. However, beyond survival rates and gross measures of mainly physical outcome (Jennett & Bond 1975), it soon became clear that measurement of outcome – and therefore measurement of the success or otherwise of interventions – was extremely complex, especially when related to the question of returning to previous life functioning.

Benefits of a holistic approach

Oddy et al (1978), Lezak (1978), Brooks and co-workers (Brooks & Aughton 1979, Brooks & McKinlay 1983) and Levin et al (1979), amongst others, began to describe various significant ongoing cognitive, social and psychological problems in different patient series. These authors brought the importance of social, cognitive and behavioural factors into focus and were successful in demonstrating that these factors, rather than physical deficits, were key in preventing individuals taking up their previous life roles in terms of relationships, home lives, and study or employment.

A number of experimental rehabilitation programmes then developed, mainly in the USA, aimed at addressing these wider issues, beyond traditional physical rehabilitation, and during the 1980s studies examining the effectiveness of specific rehabilitative programmes began to appear in the literature (Ben-Yishay et al 1985, Eames & Wood 1985, Hall & Cope 1985, Prigatano et al 1984). As well as demonstrating improved outcomes in terms of return to more active living, they also described the importance of thorough assessment, goal setting and the need for a consistent and holistic team approach. The literature has continued to reflect an ongoing emphasis on gaining a greater understanding of social, cognitive and behavioural issues.

The concept that cognitive deficits have a major impact on outcome has become more widely accepted and, as a result of the process of designing and delivering rehabilitation programmes to try to overcome these deficits (e.g. community re-entry programmes, transitional living centres and social rehabilitation programmes), a greater understanding has been gained of some of the causal relationships.

Long-term deficits

The extent to which progress has been paralleled relating to physical issues beyond the acute period is less easily assessed. Representation within the wider literature is certainly less, as is the level of representation at major conferences. It appears that in the effort to acknowledge and understand the significant impact of the less visible cognitive deficits, physical complaints and physical deficits may not have received a fair proportion of attention.

However, in a series of recent papers Hillier and colleagues in South Australia (Hillier & Metzer 1997, Hillier et al 1997a,b) question some of the received wisdom in relation to the long-term functional impact of physical complaints and deficits, their importance to individuals following TBI and whether or not there is a relatively stronger focus on physical issues where they exist alongside cognitive issues. Amongst other things, these papers describe self-reported problematic disturbance of balance in over one third of the studied TBI population 5 years postinjury and some residual upper limb deficit in one quarter. Hillier also reports a higher level of physical deficit as rated by the neurophysiotherapist when compared to individual self-report, which may indicate a similar type of underreporting that is accepted as *normal* for cognitive and behavioural issues.

Clearly much more work has to be done in this area before any conclusions can be drawn but, as a clinician with 10 years' experience of TBI in the community and as someone who sees individuals living in a variety of geographical areas in the UK, these papers have some face validity. They appear to support my own view that for many people, the potential impact of *high-level* sensorimotor dysfunction on a wide range of physical complaints and functional difficulties is not currently being considered.

Future developments

At a clinical level there is a degree of consensus in practice, primarily where the issues relate to acute management, for example respiratory care, assisting the individual to experience the normal range of antigravity positions and, to some extent, the use of seating, casting and other forms of external control or environmental adaptation. As post-acute TBI rehabilitation continues to develop, so it must include a more thorough evaluation of sensorimotor function and give due consideration to the role of less overt deficits, including their interaction with cognition and behaviour. It must be expected, given the complex nature of the central nervous system and the diffuse nature of TBI, that in dysfunction as well as in function the potential for interdependence clearly exists.

SCOPE AND STRUCTURE OF THIS BOOK

It is the inescapable interaction of the multiple systems and subsystems that underpin the functional output of the central nervous system that influences the structure and presentation of this book. The book does not attempt to follow a simple chronological progression from the acute stage onwards. Neither is the material presented in venue-specific terms. It is hoped that, although the presentation may be initially unusual to physiotherapists, the reasoning for this particular approach will soon become evident, and that if the conceptual style is new it will help the reader develop more lateral and longitudinal thinking.

SETTING THE CONTEXT

Chapters 2 and 3 are designed to set the context in terms of pathology and external influencing factors. Chapter 2 is concerned with TBI: what it is, how often it occurs and to whom. It gives an overview of common patterns of injury and the deficits associated with them, and deals briefly with the principles of acute management in relation to the prevention of secondary problems. This chapter also describes a series of potential points of contact between physiotherapists and those with TBI, and outlines the type and scope of the physiotherapist's role at each contact point.

Chapter 3 highlights the importance of seeing the person with TBI as an individual and of developing an understanding of their preinjury lifestyle, responsibilities and interests. The influence of personal history and personal characteristics on the choice of intervention design is introduced and considered alongside other major influences such as age at injury and time postinjury at the point of contact with rehabilitation services.

The impact of the trauma on family members and other involved individuals is discussed, particularly in relation to its effect on individuals' and families' abilities to respond to the demands made on them by medical and rehabilitation professionals. It is suggested within this chapter that, given the long-term nature of TBI sequelae, serious consideration should be given to the provision for families early in the history of the traumatic event and that this consideration should include the need for a flexible response to accommodate differing coping styles and social and educational backgrounds.

Finally, the influence and potential of the wider community is discussed. Within Chapter 3, and subsequently throughout the book, case examples are used to give practical illustration and make tangible links between the concepts under discussion.

ASSESSMENT

Chapters 4, 5, 6 and 7 describe the assessment process. Chapter 4 outlines the usefulness of considering a number of factors in advance of designing and undertaking the assessment. Emphasis is given to investing time in gathering previous records, in consulting previous contacts, in establishing what, if any, services are already involved and in identifying potential professional collaborators. A framework of headings is introduced to enable recording and report writing, and to raise awareness of missing knowledge where full information is not available.

The full scope of an interdisciplinary assessment process is presented in some detail in Chapters 5 and 6, with the second of these two chapters focusing on areas of assessment in which physiotherapists would expect to be directly involved. As well as describing the desired scope of the process, potential information sources and mechanisms for gathering information are also discussed.

The final part of this section, involving the setting of goals for intervention, is dealt with in Chapter 7. Topics discussed include the usefulness of cross-referencing information, negotiating with other professionals, negotiating with clients and carers, identifying priorities and the relationship between problem lists and intervention goals.

All of these chapters taken together present a mechanism for achieving good practice in the form of client-centred interdisciplinary assessment including some discussion of alternative strategies to facilitate the implementation of the underlying principles in less than ideal practice situations. Physiotherapeutic assessment of a wide range of sensorimotor and functional physical issues is addressed, and the potential for physiotherapists to contribute to the cognitive–behavioural assessment is also discussed.

INTERVENTION

The penultimate section of the book focuses on designing and delivering interventions. The first chapter in this section, Chapter 8, considers the principles of neurophysiotherapeutic practice, their evolution and present status in today's environment of evidence-based practice. An argument is developed in support of a flexible and open approach to intervention choices, and a number of ideas are floated to address the complex issues of practice development and the clinical–scientific interface.

Chapter 9 explores further the impact of the non-physical issues raised as potential influencing factors throughout the book. It attempts to promote a greater understanding of the influence of cognitive dysfunction, offering practical advice and suggesting a variety of strategies to improve direct treatment sessions and cumulative progress.

Throughout Chapter 9, and in particular within the illustrative case studies, choices of intervention and approach are also explained in terms of other individual influencing factors with the global aim of ensuring effective, relevant physical programmes. Case examples are used throughout this section to assist understanding and link relevant issues.

SERVICE PROVISION

In conclusion, the need to recognize the special service needs of the TBI population is stressed in Chapter 10. This is discussed initially in the wider context of the need to raise the profile of rehabilitation services in general and with reference to some of the issues raised by financial limitations and the impact of the relatively low status of rehabilitation compared with other areas of healthcare provision. Evidence and opinion concerning recommendations for models of care are reviewed and the discussion culminates in a suggested checklist for a model service.

CONCLUSION

In summary, this book essentially proposes a conceptual framework to assist physiotherapists to adopt a holistic approach to their contribution to rehabilitation and adjustment provision for individuals following TBI. In addition, attention is drawn to the educational and support needs of those who share their lives so that they may assist the rehabilitation process. Practical advice on physiotherapeutic intervention is given within the context of suggestions for management of other coexisting difficulties.

It is hoped that, although the text is directed primarily at physiotherapy practitioners, the philosophy and content presented will have a wider appeal and will increase awareness of the potential contribution of physiotherapists to TBI provision so that their knowledge and skills may be used to best effect.

REFERENCES

Abernethy J 1811 Surgical observations on injuries of the head and miscellaneous subjects. Dobson, Philadelphia, PA
Ben-Yishay Y, Rottock J, Lakin P et al 1985 Neuropsychologic rehabilitation: quest for a holistic approach. Seminars in Neurology 5:252–259
Brooks D, Aughton M 1979 Cognitive recovery during the first year after severe blunt head injury. International Rehabilitation Medicine 1:166–172
Brooks D, McKinlay W 1983 Personality and behavioural changes after severe blunt head injury – a relatives' view. Journal of Neurology, Neurosurgery and Psychiatry 46:336–344
Burke D 1987 Planning a system of care for head injuries. Brain Injury 1(2):189–198

Cawthorne T 1945 The physiological basis for head exercises. Journal of the Chartered Society of Physiotherapy 31:106–107

Cockburn J, Gatherer A 1988 Facilities for rehabilitation of adults after head injury. Clinical Rehabilitation 2:315–318

Cooksey F 1946 Rehabilitation in vestibular injuries. Proceedings of the Royal Society of Medicine 39:273–278

Eames P, Wood R 1985 Rehabilitation after severe brain injury: a follow-up study of a behaviour modification approach. Journal of Neurology, Neurosurgery and Psychiatry 48:613–619

Eames P, Wood R 1989 The structure and content of a head injury rehabilitation service. In: Wood R L, Eames P (eds) Models of brain injury rehabilitation, 1st edn. Chapman & Hall, London, p 31

Goldberger M, Murray M 1980 Locomotor recovery after deafferentation of one side of the cat's trunk. Experimental Neurology 67:103–117

Greenhough W T, Larson J R, Withers G S 1985 Effects of unilateral and bilateral training in a reaching task on dendritic branching or neurons in the rat motor–sensory forelimb cortex. Behavioural and Neurobiology 44:301–314

Guthrie J 1847 Injuries of the head affecting the brain. Churchill & Renshaw, London

Hall K, Cope N 1985 The current status of head injury rehabilitation. In: Millener M E, Wagner K (eds) Neurotrauma, treatment, rehabilitation and related issues. Butterworths, Boston, MA

Hillier S, Metzer J 1997 Awareness and perceptions of outcomes after traumatic brain injury. Brain Injury 11(7):525–536

Hillier S, Hiller J, Metzer J 1997a Epidemiology of traumatic brain injury in South Australia. Brain Injury 11(9):649–659

Hillier S, Sharpe M, Metzer J 1997b Outcomes 5 years post-traumatic brain injury (with further reference to neurophysical impairment and disability). Brain Injury 11(9):661–675

Hooper R 1969 Patterns of acute head injury. Edward Arnold, London

Jennett B, Bond B 1975 Assessment of outcome after severe head injury. Lancet i:480–484

Jennett B, Teasdale G 1981 Management of head injuries. FA Davis, Philadelphia, PA

Levin H, Grossman R, Rose J, Teasdale G 1979 Long term neuropsychological outcome of closed head injury. Journal of Neurosurgery 50:412–422

Lezak M 1978 Subtle sequelae of brain damage: Perplexity, distractibility and fatigue. American Journal of Physical Medicine 57:9–15

Macewen W 1881 Intracranial lesions – illustrating some points in connection with the localisation of some cerebral affections and the advantages of aseptic trephining. Lancet ii:544–551

McMillan T, Bonham E, Oddy M, Stroud A, Rickard R 1989 A comprehensive service for the rehabilitation and long-term care of head injury survivors. Clinical Rehabilitation 3:253–259

McMillan T, Greenwood R 1993 Head injury. In: Greenwood R, Barnes M P, McMillan T M, Ward C D (eds) Neurological rehabilitation, 1st edn. Churchill Livingstone, Edinburgh, p 437

Medical Disability Society 1988 The management of traumatic brain injury. The Medical Disability Society, London

Oddy M, Humphrey M, Uttley D 1978 Subjective impairment of social recovery after closed head injury. Journal of Neurology, Neurosurgery and Psychiatry 41:611–616

Prigatano G, Fordyce D, Zeiner H et al 1984 Neuropsychological rehabilitation after closed head injury in young adults. Journal of Neurology, Neurosurgery and Psychiatry 47:505–513

Teasdale G, Jennett B 1974 Assessment of coma and impaired consciousness: a practical scale. Lancet ii:81–84

Watson M 1997 Evidence for 'significant' late stage motor recovery in patients with severe traumatic brain injury: a literature review with relevance to neurological physiotherapy. Physical Therapy Review 2:93–106

Setting the context

SECTION CONTENTS

2

Understanding traumatic brain injury

Key Points

- How TBI is defined and measured
- The size and characteristics of the TBI population
- Mechanisms and types of injury
- Primary and secondary damage and the principles of acute management
- Overview of common neurodeficits and impairments
- Overview of the physiotherapeutic role throughout the course of recovery, rehabilitation and adjustment

---

INTRODUCTION

Physiotherapists may come into contact with individuals who have sustained traumatic brain injury (TBI) at varying times following injury and in varying circumstances. Whenever that professional contact takes place, whether it be during the immediate post-acute period or several years down the line, it is vital that the therapist knows and understands the severity and overall consequences of the injury.

The process of seeking out information to inform assessment after the acute period will be covered in Section 2. This chapter hopes to provide therapists with sufficient knowledge of TBI pathology to ensure understanding and accurate interpretation of medical and other early management notes.

TBI covers a wide scope of injuries and the effects of TBI are complex. The structure of this chapter is designed to give an overview of the salient knowledge that should underpin physiotherapeutic practice and will equally be of use in service planning and design.

WHAT IS TRAUMATIC BRAIN INJURY?

TBI has become the standard title used to describe what is actually a wide spectrum of subpathologies and an almost infinite variety of deficit profiles. The term *brain injury* has been adopted increasingly in preference to head injury as the importance of the site and extent of the actual *brain damage* has come more into focus. In terms of service planning and long-term outcome, it has been recognized that there is a marked difference between injuries with predominantly extracranial features and those producing intracranial disturbance. The prefix *traumatic* is added to provide a distinction from other forms of acquired brain injury such as would occur, for example, from a ruptured aneurysm.

The distinction between head injury and brain injury is particularly relevant for those who provide post-acute services in that it can reasonably be predicted that the former type of injury will produce no demand on rehabilitation services while the latter type, even in its mildest form, may require referral to those with expertise in rehabilitation or adjustment issues.

However, although this distinction may have been made in the TBI literature and has also been adopted by the majority of those specializing in the TBI field, the terms head injury, brain injury and traumatic brain injury are still used interchangeably by many healthcare professionals. It is important that physiotherapists, who may have to review medical records or gather information to inform their assessment from other documentation, are aware of the potential for this semantic confusion.

Throughout this book the term TBI is used to describe the full scope of injuries causing intracranial disruption. However, as has already been stated, this full scope comprises an extremely wide range of severity and as such it is necessary at some points to make subdivisions in terms of describing both the immediate injury and the subsequent impact on function. Therefore, it is also important for the reader to understand some of the methodological issues surrounding the assessment and recording of injury severity in the immediate and acute-care period.

HOW IS TRAUMATIC BRAIN INJURY DEFINED?

There is still no universally agreed definition of TBI. However, in an effort to emphasize TBI as a distinct entity, separate from stroke and other causes of acquired brain injury, a working party of the UK Medical Disability Society (1988, p. 3) defined TBI as:

Brain injury caused by trauma to the head (including the effects upon the brain of other possible complications of injury notably hypoxaemia and hypotension, and intracerebral haematoma).

The content in parentheses refers to the importance of recognizing the functional impact of secondary damage, the mechanisms and results of which will be discussed later in this chapter. The National Head Injury Foundation (NHIF) in the USA produced a rather more detailed definition which includes a description of resultant effects (Harrison & Dijkers 1992, p. 206):

Traumatic head injury is an insult to the brain, not of a degenerative or congenital nature but caused by an external physical force, that may produce a diminished or altered state of consciousness, which results in impairment of cognitive abilities or physical functioning. It can also result in the disturbance of behavior or emotional functioning. These impairments may be either temporary or permanent and cause partial or total functional disability or psychosocial maladjustment.

The NHIF definition is comprehensive and written in language that is easily understood. It is also inclusive of those individuals whose injuries produce only transient symptoms, encouraging the event to be recorded as a TBI and thus aiding clinical decision making should a second injury occur. This is important given the cumulative effect of repeated minor injuries (Gronwall & Wrightson 1975). However, the NHIF definition does not include any system for grading the severity of an injury and, if used, needs to be combined with other measures.

SEVERITY

The severity of TBI ranges from those who die before admission to hospital to those who do not present themselves for medical evaluation. For those who do present at emergency facilities, the type and severity of their injuries will determine immediate management and, to some extent, any subsequent intervention. The most frequently quoted indicators of severity are depth and duration of coma and/or the presence of post-traumatic amnesia. Some of the issues surrounding the assessment and documentation of these modalities will now be introduced.

COMA, ALTERED CONSCIOUSNESS AND ASSOCIATED MEASURES OF SEVERITY

The Glasgow Coma Scale

In the process of development of the Glasgow Coma Scale (GCS) (Teasdale & Jennett 1974, 1976) the authors defined coma as 'not obeying commands, not uttering words and not opening eyes'. Since its publication the GCS has become a standard assessment of altered consciousness at UK accident and emergency departments, neurosurgical departments and in many other trauma and neurosurgical centres worldwide. While the scale does have limitations and evidence of use by inadequately trained personnel has provoked questions regarding reliability (Crewe & Lye 1990, Rowley & Fielding 1991), it remains the most widely used method for assessing impaired consciousness.

The GCS comprises three subsections: eye opening, best motor response and verbal response. A completely unresponsive patient is assigned a GCS score of 3, one point for a zero response on each subsection. By the authors' definition such an individual would be deemed to be in coma and scores greater than 3 up to a summated maximum of 15 would be said to represent a varying degree of altered consciousness.

As well as being a graded measure of level of consciousness, GCS scores within the first 24 h are often regarded as indicative of the severity of the primary injury (Table 2.1). Thus, within this system, summated GCS scores between 3 and 8 are regarded as being indicative of severe injury, scores between 9 and 12 of moderate injury, and those between 13 and 15 of mild injury.

Other grading scales

Although the GCS, augmented by additional standard observations and measures, is used almost exclusively in the UK, the GCS is not the only

Table 2.1   Traumatic brain injury severity: lowest summated Glasgow Coma Score (GCS) in the first 24 h

Grade	GCS
Mild	13–15
Moderate	9–12
Severe	3–8

grading scale used to describe severity of TBI. One alternative (Najaryan 1989) is a simple scale of four definition-based grades from grade 1, 'Awake and alert, non focal neurologic examination', to grade 4, 'Without evidence of brain function or brain dead'.

While this scale, by documenting behaviour and specific evidence of neurological sequelae, appears to acknowledge the severity of an injury, each individual grade covers a wide spectrum of injuries. It is also disadvantaged by the need for a competent neurological assessment to underpin the assignation of grades. One advantage that the GCS has over this apparently more simple scale is that it has been shown to have good inter-rater reliability in trained personnel (Teasdale et al 1978) and, importantly, can be rated by trained personnel other than doctors. Both of these scales were developed from first principles based on clinical observations.

Gennarelli and colleagues (1982) developed a severity grading for TBI from experimental work with primates. They correlated neuropathological findings with previously documented clinical information to produce four grades of severity. The main neuropathological findings related to diffuse axonal injury (DAI), which will be discussed later in this chapter, and the grades of severity were based on the extent and location of the DAI and how it related to the documented clinical course from time of injury until death. The four grades reflect increasing prevalence of DAI from grade 0, no evidence of DAI/clinical concussion or mild coma, to grade 3, DAI extending to the superior cerebellar peduncle/long coma duration and poor outcome.

DURATION OF COMA OR ALTERED CONSCIOUS STATE

After the assessment of severity within the first 24 h, the second most quoted measure of severity of injury is usually the duration of coma and/or the period of altered consciousness. However, when clinicians refer to coma they may not restrict themselves to the GCS baseline of 3. Injured individuals consistently scoring 3 on the GCS are often referred to as being in deep coma, with those recording 4, 5, 6 or 7 being regarded as in coma or a severe state of altered consciousness. Bond (1990) states that 90% of those with scores of 8 or less are in coma whereas none with 9 or more are in coma.

The main purpose of briefly introducing these points of inconsistency is to alert the physiotherapist as to the need to look for specific definitions when reading published studies and to compare subjective reports in the medical notes with objective scoring, especially where subscale scores are available. By cross-referencing information in this way, therapists can establish what convention, if any, is being followed.

Table 2.2   Traumatic brain injury severity: duration of coma (GCS ≤8)

Grade	GCS
Mild	<15 min
Moderate	> 5 min, < 6 h
Severe	> 6 h, < 48 h
Very severe	> 48 h

With respect to defining severity based on length of coma or unconsciousness, a duration of less than 15 min is said to be minor, up to 6 h moderate, between 6 and 48 h severe, and greater than 48 h very severe (Table 2.2). But, as will already be obvious from the preceding commentary, these definitions may be contaminated by the inconsistent definition of coma based on summated GCS scores.

Other issues of note relate to the influence of elective ventilation, particularly when sedating or paralysing drugs are used, the influence of facial injuries preventing eye opening, that of limb fractures and specific neural deficits such as aphasia. Therefore, consideration must be given to all these factors when attempting to use coma duration as an indicator of the severity of initial injury.

As controversy remains regarding the definition of coma, so does the definition of near coma states. The term persistent vegetative state (PVS) was first coined by Jennett & Plum (1974) to describe individuals who are no longer in coma but show no evidence of higher cerebral function. The syndrome they described includes periods of wakefulness with eye opening and eye movement, and reflexive movement of the limbs but with no comprehensible speech. Even after severe injuries, most individuals open their eyes by 1 month postinjury (Bricolo et al 1980), and PVS as defined by Jennet & Plum was initially applied around this point. However, following further consideration and discussion taking into account the ethical, emotional and management impact of an individual being said to be in PVS, Berrol (1986) and others suggested the more pragmatic stance of describing the individual as being in a vegetative state but not applying the prefix 'persistent' until 12 months have elapsed from the time of injury.

It is beyond the scope of this book to enter into detailed discussion of the huge personal, ethical and societal issues raised by the emergence of individuals who survive in a severely damaged state following TBI. Therapists who become involved in the management of such individuals are referred for information to two special edition journals (Berrol & Rosenthal 1986, McMillan & Wilson 1993) and to O'Dell & Riggs (1996) and Gill-Thwaites (1997) as a starting point for further reading and consideration.

EMERGENCE FROM COMA

The documentation of emergence from coma and its potential for predicting outcome has attracted substantial attention and a number of measures have been suggested for use. This area has been a particular focus for work at Southampton University in the UK in recent years, where researchers and practitioners from many disciplines have pooled knowledge and experience creatively leading to the development of the Wessex Head Injury Matrix (WHIM).

From part of this work, Horn and colleagues (1993) produced an excellent review of a range of recovery measures. They concluded that, although the GCS remained the best overall measure in the early stages of severe injury, there was a need for more detailed behavioural observations and that those observations needed to continue beyond the period when the individual was said to be out of coma.

In this paper the authors outlined preliminary work regarding the development of a visual awareness scale, described as being part of a larger study that also looked at motor, social and communicative behaviours and other cognitive functions. Work on developing the WHIM, including reliability and validity studies and adaptations for use with children is ongoing.

The slow to recover or minimally responsive group of patients has attracted specific attention from other authors (Freeman 1996, Gill-Thwaites 1997, Wilson et al 1996), particularly in relation to the assessment of change following sensory stimulation programmes.

POST-TRAUMATIC AMNESIA

Following emergence from coma, and in some cases where coma has not occurred, there is a period during which the individual may appear confused, disoriented and/or agitated. They may confabulate and will have impaired attention. They will have difficulty recording and retrieving information concerning daily events. This period is known as the period of post-traumatic amnesia (PTA). Ritchie Russell (1932) first proposed a link between the time taken to recover full consciousness and the quantity of brain tissue destroyed, and asserted that the last stage in returning to full consciousness was demonstrated by the return of day-to-day memory on a continuous basis.

Russell defined injury severity as mild if the duration of PTA is less than 1 h, moderate if between 1 and 24 h, severe if between 1 and 7 days, and very severe if greater than 7 days (Table 2.3).

Today the term PTA is used more widely to describe the fuller package of disorientation and reduced attention outlined above. As such, attempts to assess directly the individual thought to be in PTA often include modalities other than memory. The most commonly used test is the Galveston

Table 2.3 Traumatic brain injury severity: duration of post-traumatic amnesia

Grade	GCS
Mild	< 1 h
Moderate	> 1 h, < 24 h
Severe	> 1 h, < 7 days
Very severe	> 7 days

Orientation and Amnesia Test (GOAT) (Levin et al 1979) which, in summary, measures the individual's orientation to time, person and place, and their memory for recent events. The Westmead PTA Scale (Shores et al 1986) confines itself to the measurement of amnesia and includes recognition and learning components.

The understanding of the relationship between cognition and confusion at this early stage of recovery is still limited and when therapists have access to scores produced from these or other measures of PTA they should be clear what aspects have actually been assessed and interpret the results accordingly.

In many services PTA is assessed by retrospective questioning of individuals and/or their carers. This is not without methodological difficulties; for example, Gronwall & Wrightson (1980) found that one quarter of patients changed their original estimate of PTA at a second interview 3 months later. However, it is possible to make a reasonable estimate of PTA at the level of hours, days, weeks or months via the triangulation of multiple responses and/or multiple informants. In a study comparing prospective and retrospective assessment of PTA in a population with severe TBI, McMillan and colleagues (1996) found a high correlation between the two methods and a significant correlation between severity and outcome.

It is worthy of note that, although individuals in PTA have *impaired* memory and learning abilities and may exhibit behaviours that make therapeutic interactions difficult, they are *not incapable* of all learning. There is some evidence that individuals in PTA can learn procedural tasks slowly (Ewert et al 1989, Wilson et al 1992) and that other non-verbal learning, while limited, is possible (Gasquoine 1991). This limited evidence is supportive of providing aspects of rehabilitation to those still in PTA but further work is required to define more clearly the full extent of methods that may be useful.

EPIDEMIOLOGY OF TBI

Epidemiology is the study of the incidence (number of new cases in a given population over a period of time) and prevalence (total number of existing cases within a given population at a given point in time) of a disease or condition, which allows a description of those at risk and, where possible, of what constitutes the risk. Epidemiological data can be used to estimate service needs, to plan and target preventive measures, and to assess the effect of palliative measures put in place.

Some of the issues already outlined in this chapter highlight in part the difficulties in interpreting epidemiological studies as they relate to TBI. For example, across studies various definitions of severity have been used and a variety of inclusion criteria has been applied. Some studies have included skull fractures without brain injury, some all age ranges, while others have confined themselves to adult populations.

Studies also come from substantially different healthcare systems and, even where the system is broadly the same, as in the UK, admission policies and data recording procedures vary from hospital to hospital. Existing international classification systems for disease and injury (World Health Organization 1975) include five potential codes for fractures of the face and skull and a further five codes for intracranial injuries, excluding those with fractures (Table 2.4).

Another complicating factor is that, where there are major concomitant injuries, the brain injury may not be recorded at all. It is difficult to obtain an accurate picture from routinely recorded data based on the international codes.

INCIDENCE

Having said all this, *average* incidence figures in Western developed countries derived from the range recorded in various studies based on

Table 2.4   International Classification of Diseases

Code	Description
Fracture of the skull	
800	Fracture of the vault of the skull
801	Fracture of the base of the skull
802	Fracture of the face bones
803	Other unqualified skull fractures
804	Multiple fractures involving skull or face with other bones
Intracranial injury, excluding those with skull fracture	
850	Concussion
851	Cerebral laceration and contusion
852	Subarachnoid, subdural and extradural haemorrhage, following injury
853	Other and unspecified intracranial haemorrhage, following injury
854	Intracranial injury of other and unspecified nature

presentation for medical evaluation are comparable at around 250–300 per 100 000 population. Published studies focusing on large urban areas generally produce higher incidence rates, with internal variance in causal factors related to cultural and lifestyle differences, for example high rates of assault in certain American inner-city studies.

PREVALENCE

Many of the data relating to prevalence in TBI are estimated from incidence data, taking the population age and survival rates into account. This has led to estimations of up to 439 per 100 000 (Kalsbeek et al 1980). However, a national household survey in Canada (Moscato et al 1994) produced a self-reported prevalence of disability from TBI lasting more than 6 months of only 54 per 100 000.

Bryden (1989), in an interview-based household survey of three Scottish districts, recorded a prevalence of 100 per 100 000 for those whose everyday life was affected after sustaining a TBI. Given the population mix within these three districts, Bryden argued that there is no reason why these figures should not be applicable to the rest of the UK, giving a national total of 55 000 in the late 1980s. The most recent estimate of prevalence in the UK is given at between 50 000 and 75 000 (Centre for Health Service Studies 1998).

CHARACTERISTICS OF THE TBI POPULATION
Age and gender

Whatever the overall incidence rates, certain characteristics of the adult TBI population at time of injury have proven to be consistent over many studies. The review by Sorenson & Kraus (1991) of several selected US studies is typical in showing that the highest risk of injury is between the ages of 16 and 25 years, declining until late middle age and beginning to increase again about age 60 or 65 years. This pattern of occurrence is comparable between the two sexes, although it varies in magnitude.

Kraus & McArthur (1996) described the incidence ratio between men and women as ranging between 2 : 1 and 2.8 : 1. They also made the point that the mortality rate ratio, comparing men to women, is 3.5 : 1, this being strongly indicative of more severe injuries among men. Taking these two figures together, it can be seen that in terms of TBI survivors the male : female ratio may be expected to be nearer to 2 : 1.

In the Canadian prevalence survey mentioned previously, the gender ratio is recorded as 1.8 : 1. I make this point specifically to counteract the impact of the frequently repeated statement that TBI occurs commonly in young males between the ages of 17 and 22 years. While the facts are that male survivors of TBI constitute the majority population, the needs of female survivors, being one third of a very large number, require appropriate attention. In the same way, the older TBI population requires special consideration in relation to programme design and preventive measures.

Cause of injury

In the majority of studies, transport accidents are implicated as the major cause of TBI. For example, Hillier and colleagues (1997) in South Australia reported that 57% of patients admitted to hospital with TBI in 1989 resulted from transport accidents. The same study attributed 29% of cases to falls and 9% to assaults. No subdivisions were given for the falls category in this study, nor were figures broken down to relate causal factors to age. However, males involved in transport accidents were much more likely to be the car driver (29%) than the passenger (8%), compared with rates of 24% and 22% respectively for females.

Other studies imply trends towards an increased rate of sporting accidents and falls in the younger (< 20 years) age group and towards simple falls in the older (> 60 years) age group. For example, a study focusing on an adolescent sample (Body & Leatham 1996) reported sport as the primary causal factor in males (52%) and females (76%) aged between 15 and 19 years, with transport accidents accounting for only 15% and 10% respectively. Miller & Jones (1990) reported a 77% incidence of falls in a population aged 65 years and over, and also indicated that within this population the male : female ratio is much closer to 1 : 1.

MECHANISMS AND OUTCOME OF BRAIN DAMAGE

Brain damage in TBI results from the impact on the brain tissue of the energy from the insult and from the reactive pathological processes that follow. The brain is predisposed to particular patterns of injury by nature of its structure and design, and the structure of the skull within which it is enclosed. Another factor in determining the final outcome of the injury is the preinjury status of the brain.

BRAIN STRUCTURE AND DESIGN

In understanding the mechanisms of primary injury it is worth revisiting selective aspects of anatomy and physiology. The brain consists of two large, fairly symmetrical, cerebral hemispheres below which sits, posteriorly, the smaller cerebellar structures and, centrally, the funnel of tissues which, by way of the midbrain and brainstem, eventually become the spinal cord. There are billions of differentiated cells in the brain, including the functionally important neurone. Most neurones have elongated processes called axons, which emanate from the body of the cell and carry small electrical signals or impulses. Between cells the signals are transmitted via chemical neurotransmitters and this, in simple terms, is the basis of the communication network of the brain.

The density of brain tissue differs depending on whether the area is occupied predominantly by cells (grey matter) or axons (white matter). Surrounding the brain there are three membranes, the pia mater, arachnoid mater and dura mater, known collectively as the meninges. Between the two inner membranous layers there is cerebrospinal fluid and around all of this the skull (Fig. 2.1).

There are three main points to remember when considering the effect of injuries that have movement, acceleration or deceleration as part of their process:

1. The brain is poorly anchored within the skull, allowing movement relative to the skull to occur.
2. Movement forces have a different effect on brain tissue of different densities.
3. The inside of the skull is not a smooth surface throughout.

TYPES OF INJURY

TBI often occurs without fracture of the skull; this is known as a closed injury. However, the skull can be disrupted by the nature or magnitude of the force of the injury.

Penetrating injuries

Caused by sharp and/or high-velocity foreign objects, this type of injury can cause a tract of damage as the missile passes into the brain substance. Where the velocity of penetration is high, as in gunshot wounds, the damage spreads sideways from the path of penetration. Penetrating injuries may be complicated by bone fragments, skin and hair being pushed into the brain, increasing the damage and risk of infection. The extent of observable neurological damage varies depending on the site of injury.

Local impact damage

Local impact damage can affect the scalp, the skull and the meninges as well as the brain itself. There is not always a clear relationship between the extracranial or cranial damage and the underlying brain damage as this varies with the mechanisms of the injury, particularly where the presence

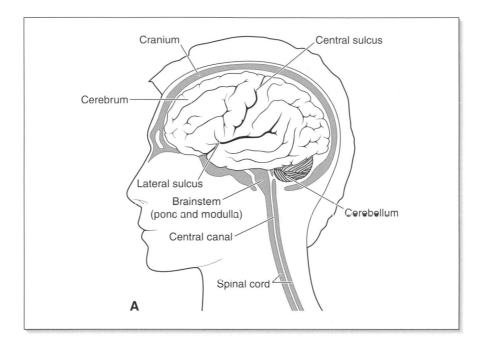

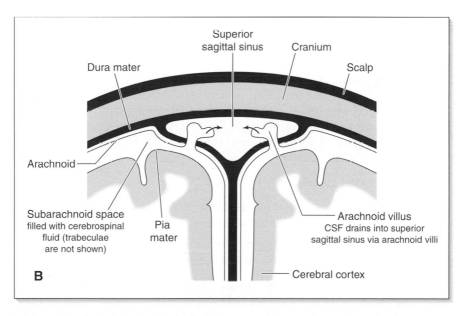

Figure 2.1 (A) Location of the brain inside the cranium. (B) Frontal section of the meninges, showing the dura mater, arachnoid and pia mater

or absence of motion is concerned. For example, a local blow with a hammer may produce a fracture with relatively little underlying brain damage, whereas the flexibility of the young skull may allow the skull to 'bend' under a more significant impact injury without breaking and yet the underlying brain tissue may be severely affected.

Skull fractures may be linear or depressed. Depressed fractures are associated with the same increased risk factors outlined under penetrating injuries. However, about half are reported to occur without loss, or with only momentary loss, of consciousness (Miller & Jennett 1968), indicating that substantial diffuse injury has not occurred.

Linear fractures may be associated with intracranial bleeding which, if left, may collect, producing a mass effect (see Secondary damage below) on the underlying brain. Local contusions or lacerations may be produced in the cerebral cortex and, where extensive, may be also associated with an intracranial collection of blood.

Polar and other internal impact damage

Depending on the site of impact and the energy involved in the insult, cortical contusions and lacerations may be produced in areas other than those directly under the area of impact. This effect is dependent on the head being subjected to acceleration or deceleration and also on the brain's ability to move relative to the skull as a result of the poor anchorage mentioned above.

When the movement is suddenly stopped, damage may occur at the opposite pole via a rebound effect (e.g. frontal damage in an occipital impact injury) and in cortical areas adjacent to the internal areas of the skull that are irregular in form. Thus, contusions are commonly found on the undersurface of the temporal and frontal lobes and on the anterior poles of the temporal lobes, regardless of the site of impact. Because of the particular design of the irregularities, occipital impacts produce more of these shearing contusions than frontal impacts.

Diffuse axonal damage

An additional consequence of the movement potential of the brain within the cranium is the production of shearing forces, which result in axons being stretched or severed within their myelin sheaths (Adams et al 1977). This is known as diffuse axonal injury (DAI), and when it is widespread it is associated with severe injury.

Mild stretch injury is thought to be responsible for transient changes in conscious level often referred to as concussion, but since this damage is not visible on computed tomography it has been difficult to produce objective evidence. With the advent of magnetic resonance imaging, some objective evidence of physical damage in relatively mild injury has begun to be recorded (Yokota et al 1991).

Other primary damage

Impact or shearing forces, or penetrating foreign bodies, may also lead to direct damage of blood vessels. Where this damage is significant, the effects are obvious immediately. However, relatively minor tears can lead to a slower accumulation of an intracranial collection and this is a particular reason for vigilance in the hours immediately after an injury that is not initially regarded as severe.

SECONDARY DAMAGE

Secondary damage is caused by the pathological process that begins with the injury itself along with the effects of aggressive secondary factors such as the mechanical effects of raised intracranial pressure, the disease process associated with infection or complications brought about by systemic dysfunction. The systemic dysfunction may be a result of the brain damage itself or it may result from concomitant injuries sustained at the same time as the brain injury.

Brain distortion and herniation

One of the most easily understood processes of secondary damage is related to the distortion caused by expanding masses or rising pressure within the cranium. When a collection of blood (haematoma) gathers, the underlying brain is distorted, initially moving to take up space normally occupied by cerebrospinal fluid. If the process continues, the affected hemisphere protrudes into adjacent intracranial compartments. This may lead to the occlusion of major arteries and/or a pattern of progressive neurological deficits as measured by the GCS. The same pattern can occur in the absence of haematoma when the brain mass is increased by congestive and/or oedematous processes such that progressive impingement of the same vital structures results.

Biochemical damage

Dead, dying and dysfunctional cells are unable to transfer or absorb water in the normal way and local oedema may occur. Ischaemic brain tissues also release substances that can cause damage to adjacent, initially uninjured areas, adding to the resultant neurological deficit. The production of a drug to limit this cascading process of damage is at present an area of intense research.

MANAGEMENT

ISSUES IN ACUTE MANAGEMENT

Factors affecting cerebral blood flow

In normal circumstances a process known as *cerebral autoregulation* (Aitkenhead 1986) ensures that blood flow to the brain is consistently maintained independent of normal fluctuations in systemic blood pressure. This is important because the energy requirements of the brain are extremely high and there is no facility for energy storage locally. The injured brain loses the autoregulation function and the blood flow or cerebral perfusion pressure (CPP) becomes directly related to the systemic mean arterial blood pressure (MABP) and the intracranial pressure (ICP). In these circumstances CPP = MABP – ICP.

A second physiological mechanism influencing cerebral blood flow is the *intracranial pressure–volume response*. This is based on a degree of flexibility within the fluid systems in the cranium, which allows for variations in the brain tissue volume. If brain tissue volume begins to increase, CSF absorption also increases and there is a secondary response in the venous system, which reduces the cerebral blood volume. However, when these mechanisms are exhausted, any further small increase in the volume is accompanied by an increase in ICP (Fig. 2.2).

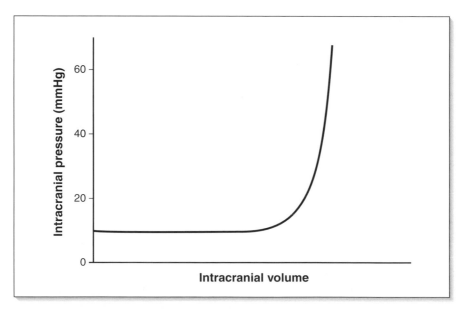

Figure 2.2   Relationship between intracranial volume and intracranial pressure

Normally, ICP in the supine position is in the region of 0–10 mmHg and a sustained pressure greater than 20 mmHg is regarded as abnormal. ICP is abnormally high in 70% of serious injuries (Bullock & Teasdale 1990), indicating that the normal pressure–volume response has been exceeded. As ICP rises, the CPP decreases, reducing the delivery of oxygen at a time when the brain has increased energy requirements (Frost 1985).

Hypoxaemia

A reduced level of oxygen in the blood after TBI may be attributed to the brain injury or may result from pulmonary complications (Gentleman et al 1993), and has been noted in more than one third of severely injured patients on arrival at hospital (Miller et al 1981). In normal circumstances the response to oxygen desaturation of arterial blood would be cerebral vasodilatation. This response is reduced or absent in the damaged brain and is another factor, along with those already outlined, that contributes to poor oxygenation of the injured brain.

Thus, the injury to the brain itself removes a number of the body's protective compensatory mechanisms necessitating intensive medical management to limit further insult to the already damaged brain. The management of all of these interrelated issues is one of the key factors in successful acute management, and the concept of managing preventable secondary effects can be recognized in all good practice throughout acute management and beyond.

SUMMARY OF THE PRINCIPLES OF ACUTE MANAGEMENT

Evaluation and stabilization

Paramedic and other emergency services staff have established guidelines for the management of TBI in the acute stage based on providing the best conditions for recovery from any primary brain damage and preventing complications that lead to secondary brain damage. The role of the accident and emergency department is summarized in an article by Bullock & Teasdale (1990) which reviews good practice in the management of acute TBI as follows:

- Resuscitate, diagnose, and record
- Detect or exclude other injuries
- Request, supervise and interpret results of radiography and other initial investigations
- Decide whether admission is needed and, if so, where
- Liaise with other specialties (e.g. neurosurgery) about serious cases
- Ensure adequate arrangements for observing and maintaining the patient's condition during transfer to other departments or hospitals

- Observe the progress of patients with minor injuries, who should be admitted to short-stay beds
- Ensure adequate arrangements for follow-up.

The primary objectives are to establish and maintain a clear airway with appropriate oxygenation and to maintain an adequate peripheral circulation via an adequate blood volume. With these aspects under control, accurate neurological assessment can be made. Particular care is always taken to limit movement of the cervical spine until fracture has been excluded. Investigations are performed only when this baseline status has been achieved and thoroughly documented. Prophylactic antibiotic and anticonvulsant therapy is commenced in at-risk patients.

Neurosurgical intervention

Surgery is undertaken to decompress the brain, for example in the presence of a large haematoma, or to perform debridement and lavage of compound fracture wounds to help prevent infection. In some centres surgery is performed to insert a device for monitoring the ICP in a subpopulation of severely injured patients or in those with associated face and/or chest injuries.

Limitation of secondary brain damage

Adequate oxygenation

Assisted respiration in the form of ventilation is provided for all patients who exhibit abnormal respiration. In many centres elective ventilation is used for the first three days in all severe injuries and when there are associated facial, abdominal and/or chest injuries. Ventilated patients are usually also sedated and paralysed, and this has additional management effects. Combined, they result in a reduction in cerebral blood volume, and breathing patterns can be set to manipulate blood gas (oxygen and carbon dioxide) levels artificially, as appropriate to the individual's condition.

Ventilation is usually achieved via an endotracheal tube with tracheostomy being performed only in particular circumstances, for example when there are facial or spinal fractures or when, for reasons of injury severity or pulmonary dysfunction, ventilation is required for a protracted period.

In moderate injuries, when ventilation is not required, oxygen therapy is still advised to meet the injured brain's increased requirements.

Controlling intracranial pressure

In addition to the management of blood gases and blood volume, it is sometimes necessary to apply additional management principles and drug therapies. The patient is positioned in a head-up, but not forward flexed, position to compensate for the lack of valves in the cerebral venous system, and activities and interventions that produce an increase in ICP are minimized. ICP will increase if there is pressure on the jugular veins, hence the avoidance of neck flexion; it is also adversely affected by any increase in intrathoracic pressure, for example coughing or during manual hyper-inflation procedures. This has obvious implications for the design of physiotherapeutic intervention.

Drug selection is based on whether the desired method of management is to reduce true cerebral oedema or to reduce congestion by decreasing cerebral blood flow.

General care

Patients with TBI require the same high standard of care from the full hospital team as any other ill or injured patient. It is not within the scope of this book to deal with the acute management of all the possible associ-ated injuries and medical complications that may coexist with TBI. It is noted, however, that about 40% of severely injured patients will have other injuries (Gentleman et al 1986) whose management will need to be coordinated with that of the brain injury.

In general, medical management is prioritized in terms of the threat to life. However, beyond the need to preserve life, the specialist nature of the care and rehabilitation required by those who have sustained a TBI should mean early transfer to a treating facility with TBI expertise.

It is not possible to clearly separate the description of acute management from the often parallel process of prevention of secondary complications. However, some important principles of wider management are mentioned for completeness.

Environmental control

The environment around the injured individual can be manipulated for positive effect. Temperature, noise and activity levels are among a wide variety of factors that may be controlled. For example, hypothermia may be used to aid the management of dangerous increases in temperature that may coexist with decerebrate posturing.

Nutrition

Nutritional requirements increase after TBI and are further raised in the presence of multiple injuries such as long bone fractures. In severe injuries, the immediate postinjury phase is concerned with fluid balance manage-ment and then with establishing that gastric absorption is present.

Nutrition will then be supplied via a nasogastric tube or, in an increasing number of centres, via a gastrostomy or jejunostomy.

Adequate nutrition is essential for the maintenance of healthy body tissues as well as for healing. Vitamins E, C and A are said to limit the formation of free radicals, the accelerated production of which is part of the process of secondary brain damage.

Positioning

Positioning, assisted movement and immobilization may all be used to influence immediate and longer-term cosmetic and functional outcome in the musculoskeletal system. In the early acute phase these modalities are used to prevent complications that may be anticipated from the individual's medical and neurological status. The primary aim is to promote the optimum circumstances for recovery by working for the maintenance of balanced muscle length and extensibility around each joint and body part.

Respiratory care

As in the immediate period following injury, maintenance of a good oxygenated blood supply is crucial to the ideal of promoting optimal conditions for healing and recovery. Neurological depression of respiratory function, abnormal breathing patterns, immobility, increased risk of infection and local injury are all potential threats to the respiratory system. All members of the care team should be involved in the process of limiting the threats to respiratory health by careful observation and appropriate intervention.

Common neurological deficits and continuing impairments

The term *neurological deficit* is another example of a term that does not necessarily mean the same thing to all health professionals. For some it applies to any deficit of which the origin can be traced back to central or peripheral nervous system damage. Others would state that an individual has no neurological deficit if examination of the motor and sensory system including the cranial nerves did not reveal any problems, even though a psychometric assessment of the same individual, such as would be performed by a neuropsychologist, may well unmask deficits, for example of memory or of planning skills.

In terms of observable deficits or ongoing impairments following TBI, few are clearly apparent in the acute stage and a number of others can be confirmed only by specific testing or structured observation in a functional setting. For this reason, the description below is divided into primary, secondary and tertiary phases, and it is important to note that ongoing evaluation is essential to obtain an accurate assessment of the true level of impairment.

The extent and severity of deficits affecting each individual will obviously vary to a great extent and the deficits outlined here are primarily representative of those presenting potential challenges to therapeutic management or in the delivery of therapeutic intervention.

Primary phase

Other than the changes in conscious level, the most obvious results of central nervous system damage in the primary phase are those of motor behaviour. In addition to the best (motor) scores recorded via use of the GCS, the behaviour or responses of the other limbs, the trunk and eyes can give an indication of the extent of the damage and, in some cases, the likelihood of continuing motor deficit.

While severe injuries are commonly accompanied by raised tone, flaccid limbs may indicate additional sites of injury, for example spinal cord, brachial plexus or peripheral nerve. Spinal cord injury is said to occur in 4% of severe TBIs, while spinal cord injury has been reported as having associated mild TBI in between 25% and 50% of cases (Narayan et al 1990).

Imbalances in muscle activity or absence of activity can quickly lead to secondary soft tissue changes. Antigravity muscles appear to be most at risk and a number of other factors, such as disuse, resting muscle length and the frequency of stretch, have been identified as important parameters in preventive management (Goldspink & Williams 1990).

Secondary phase

As the period of acute illness or depressed consciousness comes to an end, more accurate assessment of a number of potential deficits becomes possible. Thus, cranial nerve function should be checked and a more detailed assessment of sensorimotor function carried out.

Olfaction.   The sense of smell is frequently lost or impaired following TBI; this may be at a primary detection level or at the level of perception or discrimination of aromas. Olfactory nerve damage is often the result of shearing damage at the cribriform plate or found in association with anterior fossa fractures.

Vision.   The visual system may be affected via direct or ischaemic damage to the optic nerve or via damage to other cerebral structures involved in the processing or interpretation of visual stimuli. Eye movements may be disrupted by damage to the oculomotor, trochlear or abducens nerves, and may be observed by the assessor as strabismus (malalignment) or reported by the patient as diplopia (double vision). Damage to the oculomotor nerve can also lead to difficulties with pupillary control and light accommodation.

Facial nerves.   Trigeminal nerve damage occurs with facial fractures and may lead to facial numbness or hypersensitivity. The facial nerve may be damaged extracranially in the preauricular area or in association with temporal fracture. The latter may present as a delayed palsy from pressure associated with swelling in the restrictive bony canal; this type carries a more positive recovery outcome.

Hearing and balance.   Damage to the vestibulocochlear nerve and its functional apparatus is also associated with temporal impact and fracture. Neural deafness may occur as a result of nerve damage, and conduction deafness as a result of dislocation of the bony chain or bleeding into the middle ear. Vestibular function may also be disrupted by local damage to the vestibular apparatus, by the creation of a perilymph fistula or by an occurrence known as labyrinthine concussion, which may also occur with some occipital impacts.

Lower cranial nerves.   The incidence of lower cranial nerve trauma, as opposed to dysfunction associated with brainstem damage, is said to be minimal, although it is acknowledged that some injuries may occur with occipital/basal fracture or in association with neck trauma.

Neck trauma.   The question of the contribution of neck trauma to TBI symptomatologies, especially in mild TBI or in the presence of suspected post-traumatic stress disorder, is beginning to be addressed in the literature (Couch 1995, Gerber & Schraa 1995, Parker 1996, Taylor et al 1996), although it is far from clear what, if any, relationship will be identified in either direction. There is no doubt, however, that the mechanical forces involved in TBI are related to those causing bony spinal trauma, and it can be assumed that there are cases where the forces involved fall short of producing fracture but do cause damage to other tissues.

It is accepted that traumatic transection of the carotid or vertebral arteries, although infrequent, does occur. In addition, in a paper presented to an international brain injury conference in Melbourne, Nathan Zasler (1996) reported a 38% incidence of abnormal cervical examination in a series of 300 outpatients with TBI, including four with previously undiagnosed disc herniation. It may be that, in the early stages of recovery, headache of cervical origin is difficult to differentiate from that resulting from other causes, or possibly has yet to develop or is not perceived or reported due to disturbed cognitive processes.

Movement disorders.   Depending on the site of injury a variety of distinct or combined motor disorders may begin to be recognized during this secondary stage. As well as the more common hypertonicity and ataxias, dyskinesias, tremors or other involuntary movements may also develop. However, these less common movement disorders appear, in some cases, to have a latent period before they are clearly recognizable.

Sensory impairment. As well as the sensory deficits discussed in relation to cranial nerve damage, a variety of central and peripheral sensory impairments may be present. These can include difficulties with the perception or interpretation of visual, tactile or proprioceptive information, or disturbance within the sensorimotor loop, for example dyspraxia.

Language. Communication problems may be expected in the early recovery phase. They may be a secondary result of cognitive blunting, due to linguistic failure as a direct result of focal or vascular injury, or due to difficulties in speech production associated with other motor deficits including dysphagia. Again, it can be difficult to differentiate between linguistic and other cognitive reasons for poor language function at this stage, as formal assessment may not be feasible. However, as agitated and confused behaviour recedes, limited testing to inform therapeutic intervention can begin.

Tertiary phase

Motor deficits may be clearly evident from the point of injury and, particularly in specialist centres, active management will often commence before medical stability is achieved. Other consequences, most notably continuing cognitive and behavioural sequelae, may not begin to be quantified for some weeks or months after moderate or severe injury, and the full extent of their functional impact, even after minor injury, cannot be ascertained until a full return to preinjury activities is attempted.

Some of the confounding factors in relation to the timing of assessment and intervention regarding these issues are discussed in more detail in Chapter 3 and their potential impact on physical intervention or physical management programmes are discussed in Chapter 9.

Cognitive and behavioural deficits. Complaints of mental fatigue and limitations of concentration are extremely common. A variety of attentional disorders may persist (see Ch. 5) and, even where recovery is good, a limitation in the speed of information processing often remains. A variety of deficits of memory and learning are encountered beyond the period of post-traumatic amnesia, affecting visual or verbal recall, or both.

A whole range of advanced cognitive and mature behavioural functions associated with frontal lobe damage may also be present, affecting the ability to think in a reasoned or creative way, to plan or act with due regard to past experience or likely future consequences, or to behave in a socially appropriate or sensitive way.

Not all people who sustain TBI have all of these difficulties but the frequency of frontal and temporal lobe damage makes the occurrence of impairment of these and other functions dependent on the integrity of these areas of the brain, such as motivation, commonplace in the TBI population. Specific behavioural syndromes, for example episodic dyscontrol which is sometimes associated with temporal lobe epilepsy, may also occur, as well as a number of reactive disturbances of mood and behaviour.

Epilepsy.   Post-traumatic epilepsy is an accepted potential consequence of TBI. The incidence of late epilepsy (i.e. after the first week following trauma) has been reported as between 2.5% and 5% (Jennett 1990) and, although more than half will begin having seizures within the first year, around one quarter start to experience epilepsy after more than 4 years postinjury.

Individuals may develop any form of epilepsy including full grand mal seizures or a variety of forms of temporal lobe epilepsy such as absences, so called psychic phenomena, such as olfactory hallucinations, *déjà vu* or physical nausea, or repetitive ritualistic behaviours known as automatisms. Temporal lobe seizures may not initially be recognized as epilepsy, and not all cases are accompanied by positive electroencephalographic recordings. However, suspected cases may respond well to a trial of anti-convulsant therapy.

Other complications.   Other medical complications may develop as a direct consequence of brain damage. For example, a variety of hormonal imbalances can result from damage to the hypothalamus or pituitary stalk, and these may present as problems only a substantial time after injury.

The potential for physiotherapeutic intervention

At all stages in TBI rehabilitation, our role as physiotherapists should be defined as part of a team and extended to include education and information giving for the friends and family of the injured person. The physio-therapist is without question a valued and valuable member of the acute care team, contributing to respiratory health and physical management of the unconscious patient.

It is essential that our direct practice, even in acute care, is always balanced by adopting a sufficiently wide perspective to include effective delivery of care by the whole team, resulting in interventions that are respectful of the injured person's individuality. It is not common practice for therapists to seek formal permission to intervene in acute care and, while as an inpatient the individual's care remains the responsibility of the medical practitioner, the vulnerability of the cognitively impaired patient and the resultant additional responsibilities that we as professionals then carry should not be overlooked.

With our knowledge of the potential long-term negative effects of poor or short-sighted early management, we have a responsibility to monitor the physical aspects of acute management and promote informed developments in practice in line with emerging evidence. In practice, this means developing an ongoing awareness of the literature, frequent close liaison and often joint working with other treating professionals, and it also means being able to accept and to give advice as appropriate to specialist knowledge.

Within subacute provision, the physiotherapeutic role usually revolves around working with those with major physical deficits or assisting individuals to achieve primary functional goals. Where contact is over a longer period of time, there is the additional opportunity to address more subtle physical limitations, or issues relating to stamina and conditioning, in preparation for a return to a wider range of life activities.

Physiotherapeutic provision should always have an end goal that improves the quality or scope of physical activity, maintains function or limits physical deterioration. Often, interventions and end goals in the acute and the early subacute phase are almost predetermined by the medical status or immediate self-care needs of the individual. Active consideration of which category of end goal it is most relevant to focus on becomes much more of a live issue when an individual has returned home or has been placed in some sort of community-based provision.

Planned physiotherapeutic provision for community-based individuals has been slow to develop for many reasons. There is, for example, an overall lack of post-acute provision. It is also still frequently asserted that no significant physical change can occur beyond 6 months after the injury. In addition, the emphasis within specialist independent services has continued to focus on social, cognitive and behavioural rehabilitation, which was originally a response to the complete lack of recognition of the need to address these issues within traditional healthcare provision. Therefore, whereas approaches to remediate or compensate for changes in cognition and behaviour have received growing attention within the literature, and functional outcome is increasingly being assessed in terms of social and community integration, the level of documentation and understanding of physical issues and their contribution to overall outcome has barely progressed beyond whether someone can walk and, if so, whether they use an aid to do so.

With particular reference to the issue of evidence of efficacy, and to quote the title of a well argued article published in the *British Medical Journal*, 'Absence of evidence is not evidence of absence' (Bland & Altmand 1995), clinical experience has taught me that specific change in physical skills and meaningful change in functional abilities can certainly be achieved well beyond the 6-month cutoff when physical intervention is delivered as part of a planned global approach, which takes into account coexisting deficits and social issues. And, in the longer term, function and quality of life can be preserved or improved by the proactive management of the effects of residual motor and sensory deficits.

These personal assertions obviously require the backup of formal audit and research activities, as does the whole process of rehabilitation and management following TBI. First, however, a standard of provision and some consistency of practice within that provision are necessary.

CONCLUSION

The TBI population is not a homogeneous group in terms of severity, deficit, age, gender or social background, and local cultural issues relating to cause and population profile also need to be taken into account in the planning of services and educational programmes or campaigns. However, there are certain undeniable facts and informative messages that emanate from examination of the issues outlined in this chapter.

A great many people sustain one or more TBIs in their lifetime, a substantial proportion in childhood, adolescent or early adult years. While this book makes no attempt to focus on the specific immediate rehabilitation needs of children, it does recognize that all children who survive eventually become adults whose needs will have to be met by adult services. Given the skewed age of the population, the cumulative prevalence of TBI survivors in societies with sophisticated healthcare provision is still increasing. This will be accompanied by increasing demands on services and will present additional issues when there are greater numbers of survivors within the elder population.

It is not yet possible to predict, at the time of injury or in the immediate subacute phase, what the functional outcome for the injured individual will be. Indeed, a number of specific deficits may not be apparent or confirmed until long after the person has been discharged from inpatient care. However, there are recognizable gross patterns of deficits across the population as a whole that allow anticipation of potential deficits and their probable functional impact. If this predictable deficit profile is combined with our knowledge of the numbers likely to be involved, it should be possible to design a matrix around which to develop appropriate service provision.

In addition, as we shall see in the next chapter, TBI does not impact only on the individual who sustains the injury. It is of extreme importance, therefore, that in recognizing the lifelong impact on the individual and the implications for service provision we should also consider the impact on, and potential contribution of, family and other potential support systems.

REFERENCES

Adams J, Mitchell D, Graham D et al 1977 Diffuse brain damage of the immediate impact type. Brain 100:489–502
Aitkenhead A 1986 Cerebral protection. British Journal of Hospital Medicine 35:290–298
Berrol S 1986 Evolution and the persistent vegetative state. Journal of Head Trauma Rehabilitation 1(1):7–13
Berrol S, Rosenthal M (eds) 1986 The persistent vegetative state. Journal of Head Trauma Rehabilitation 1(1).

Bland J M, Altmand D G 1995 Absence of evidence is not evidence of absence. British Medical Journal 311:485

Body C, Leatham J 1996 Incidence and aetiology of head injury in a New Zealand adolescent sample. Brain Injury 10(8):567–573

Bond R 1990 Standardised methods for assessing and predicting outcome. In: Rosenthal M, Griffith E, Bond M, Miller J (eds) Rehabilitation of the adult and child with traumatic brain injury, 2nd edn. FA Davis, Philadelphia, PA

Bricolo A, Turazzi S, Feriotti G 1980 Prolonged post-traumatic unconsciousness. Therapeutic assets and liabilities. Journal of Neurology, Neurosurgery and Psychiatry 52:625–634

Bryden J 1989 How many head-injured? In: Wood R, Eames P (eds) Models of brain injury rehabilitation. Chapman & Hall, London, p 17

Bullock R, Teasdale G 1990 Head injuries –1. British Medical Journal 300:1515–1518

Centre for Health Service Studies 1998 National Traumatic Brain Injury Study. Warwick University, Warwick, UK

Couch J R 1995 Post-concussion syndrome. Journal of Neurological Rehabilitation 9(2):83–89

Crewe H, Lye R 1990 Nurses' knowledge of coma assessment. Nursing Times 86:52–53

Ewert J, Levin H, Watson M, Kalisky Z 1989 Procedural memory during posttraumatic amnesia in survivors of severe closed head injury: implications for rehabilitation. Archives of Neurology 46:911–916

Freeman E 1996 The Coma Exit Chart: assessing the patient in prolonged coma and the vegetative state. Brain Injury 10(8):615–624

Frost E A M 1985 Management of head injury. Canadian Anaesthetic Society Journal 32(3):532

Gasquoine P 1991 Learning in post-traumatic amnesia following extremely severe closed head injury. Brain Injury 5(2):169–175

Gennarelli T, Thibault L, Adams J et al 1982 Diffuse axonal injury and traumatic coma in the primate. Annals of Neurology 12:564–574

Gentleman D, Teasdale G, Murray L 1986 Cause of severe head injury and risk of complications. British Medical Journal 292:449

Gentleman D, Dearden M, Midgley S, Maclean D 1993 Guidelines for resuscitation and transfer of patients with serious head injury. British Medical Journal 307:547–552

Gerber D J, Schraa J C 1995 Mild traumatic brain injury: searching for the syndrome. Journal of Head Trauma Rehabilitation 10(4):28–40

Gill-Thwaites H 1997 The sensory modality assessment rehabilitation technique – a tool for assessment and treatment of patients with severe brain injury in a vegetative state. Brain Injury 11(10):723–734

Goldspink G, Williams P 1990 Muscle fibre changes and connective tissue changes associated with use and disuse. In: Ada L, Canning C (eds) Key issues in neurological physiotherapy, 1st edn. Butterworth–Heinemann, London, p 197

Gronwall D, Wrightson P 1975 Cumulative effect of concussion. Lancet ii:995–997

Gronwall D, Wrightson P 1980 Duration of post-traumatic amnesia after mild head injury. Journal of Clinical Neuropsychology 2:51–60

Harrison C L, Dijkers M 1992 Traumatic brain injury registries in the United States: an overview. Brain Injury 6:203–212

Hillier S, Hiller J, Metzer J 1997 Epidemiology of traumatic brain injury in South Australia. Brain Injury 11(9):649–659

Horn S, Sheil A, McLellan L, Campbell M, Watson M, Wilson B 1993 A review of behavioural assessment scales for monitoring recovery in and after coma with pilot data on a new scale of visual awareness. Neuropsychological Rehabilitation 3(2):121–137

Jennett B 1990 Post-traumatic epilepsy. In: Rosenthal M, Griffith E R, Bond M R, Miller J D (eds) Rehabilitation of the adult and child with traumatic brain injury, 2nd edn. FA Davis, Philadelphia, PA, p 89

Jennett B, Plum F 1974 Persistent vegetative state after brain damage: a syndrome in search of a name. Lancet i:734–737

Kalsbeek W, McLaurin R, Harris B, Miller J 1980 The national head and spinal cord survey: major findings. Journal of Neurosurgery 53:19–31

Kraus J F, McArthur D L 1996 Epidemiological aspects of brain injury. Neurological Clinics 14(2):435–450

Levin H, O'Donnell V, Grossman R 1979 The Galveston Orientation and Amnesia Test: a practical scale to assess cognition after head injury. Journal of Nervous and Mental Diseases 167:675–684

McMillan T, Wilson S (eds) 1993 Coma and the persistent vegetative state. Neuropsychological Rehabilitation 3(2)

McMillan T, Jongen E, Greenwood R 1996 Assessment of post-traumatic amnesia after severe closed head injury: retrospective or prospective? Journal of Neurology, Neurosurgery and Psychiatry 60(4):422–427

Medical Disability Society 1988 The management of traumatic brain injury. Medical Disability Society, London

Miller J, Butterworth J F, Gudeman S K et al 1981 Further experience in the management of severe head injury. Journal of Neurosurgery 54:289

Miller J, Jennett B 1968 Complications of depressed skull fractures. Lancet ii:991–995

Miller J, Jones P 1990 Minor head injury. In: Rosenthal M, Griffith E, Bond M, Miller J (eds) Rehabilitation of the adult and child with traumatic brain injury, 2nd edn. FA Davis, Philadelphia, PA, p 236

Moscato B, Trevisan M, Willer B 1994 The prevalence of traumatic brain injury and co-occurring disabilities in a national household survey of adults. Journal of Neuropsychiatry and Clinical Neurosciences 6:134–142

Najaryan R 1989 Emergency room management of the head injured patient. In: Becker D, Gudeman S (eds) Textbook of head injury. WB Saunders, Philadelphia, PA, p 24

Narayan R K, Gokaslan Z L, Bontke C F, Berrol S 1990 Neurologic sequelae of head injury. In: Rosenthal M, Griffith E R, Bond M R, Miller J D (eds) Rehabilitation of the adult and child with traumatic brain injury, 2nd edn. FA Davis, Philadelphia, PA, p 94

O'Dell M, Riggs R 1996 Management of the minimally responsive patient. In: Horn L, Zasler N (eds) Medical rehabilitation of traumatic brain injury, 1st edn. Hanley & Belfus, Philadelphia, PA, p 103

Parker R S 1996 A taxonomy of neurobehavioural functions applied to neuropsychological assessment after head injury. Neuropsychology Review 6(3):135–170

Rowley G, Fielding K 1991 Reliability and accuracy of the Glasgow Coma Scale with experienced and inexperienced users. Lancet 337:535–538

Russell W 1932 Cerebral involvement in head injury. Brain 55:549–603

Shores E, Marosszeky J, Sandanam L, Batchelor J 1986 Preliminary validation of a scale for measuring the duration of post-traumatic amnesia. Medical Journal of Australia 144:569–573

Sorenson S B, Kraus J F 1991 Occurrence, severity, and outcomes of brain injury. Journal of Head Trauma Rehabilitation 6(2):1–10

Taylor A E, Cox C A, Mailis A M 1996 Persistent neuropsychological deficits following whiplash: evidence for chronic mild traumatic brain injury? Archives of Physical Medicine and Rehabilitation 77:529–535

Teasdale G, Jennett B 1974 Assessment of coma and impaired consciousness: a practical scale. Lancet ii:81–84

Teasdale G, Jennett B 1976 Assessment and prognosis of coma after head injury. Acta Neurochirurgica 34:45–55

Teasdale G, Knill-Jone R, van der Sande J 1978 Observer variability in assessing impaired consciousness and coma. Journal of Neurology, Neurosurgery and Psychiatry 41:603–610

Wilson B, Baddeley A, Sheil A, Patton G 1992 How does post-traumatic amnesia differ from the amnesic syndrome and from chronic memory impairment? Neuropsychological Rehabilitation 2:231–243

Wilson S, Brock G, Powell G, Thwaites H, Elliot K 1996 Constructing arousal profiles for vegetative patients – a preliminary report. Brain Injury 10(2):105–113

World Health Organization 1975 Manual of the international statistical classification of diseases, injuries and causes of death. WHO, Geneva

Yokota H, Kurokawa A, Otsuka T et al 1991 Significance of magnetic resonance imaging in acute head injury. Journal of Trauma 31:351–357

Zasler N 1996 Cervical somatic dysfunction: incidence as a factor in post-concussive headache. Australian Academic Press, Melbourne

3

Understanding the impact of the traumatic event and the influence of life context

Key Points

- The impact of TBI spreads far beyond the injured person
- The experience of each person who is affected by TBI differs in some detail but patterns of response are recognizable and can assist the development of management plans
- Accurate, consistently presented, accessible information is crucial at all stages of service contact
- Intervention and management plans must be culturally relevant
- Intervention and management goals must reflect the essence of the injured person
- Professionals must adopt a wide perspective and a longitudinal view within their local decision-making activities

INTRODUCTION

Neurophysiotherapists are specialists in the assessment and physical treatment of movement disorders. Their primary focus is in identifying the neuromuscular, sensory and biomechanical factors contributing to a particular individual's movement disorder and in applying physical interventions and management principles to improve or maintain physical function or to retard deterioration. However, physiotherapists also regard themselves as holistic practitioners and acknowledge the potential influence of wider factors on the success or otherwise of their therapeutic interventions.

It has already been stated that the rehabilitation approach outlined in this book is one that attempts to place the injured individual and those directly affected by the outcome of the traumatic event at the centre of the process. This principle is adopted so that the process of rehabilitation is relevant and timely, and the outcome of rehabilitation is meaningful for the individual concerned.

If this approach is to be achieved, the therapeutic team must develop some understanding of all the individuals with whom they need to work: who they are, where they come from, and what strengths and limitations they may have. This knowledge is gained from the assessment process and from placing the findings of that process in the context of wider knowledge established from previous academic and clinical work.

The practicalities of the assessment process that supports this approach and the potential role of physiotherapists within that process are covered in detail in Section 2. This chapter is not concerned with defining responsibility for collecting specific aspects of information but with establishing a basic understanding of the predictable impact of the traumatic event on the injured individual and on their friends and families. It asks therapists to consider contributory factors that may influence carer reactions, such as past family history or operational style, and how programme design and outcome may be further influenced by cultural or other wider community factors.

There are two primary intentions in directing therapists to consider the need to have knowledge of these wider issues. The first relates to providing what might be called a user-friendly service, that is, one that feels comfortable and relevant to those accessing it. The second relates to therapist satisfaction, both in terms of ease of service delivery and in terms of positive progress towards therapeutic goals and good functional outcome.

In short, it is asserted that if therapists understand key aspects of their client's lifestyle, have knowledge of the process that they and their families are going through and how they as therapists can help or hinder their progress, then the service they provide will feel appropriate to those they serve and will be proven relevant by the achievement of acceptable functional progress. Working in this way reduces the potential for conflict between professionals and service users, allowing maximum energy to be channelled into achieving positive therapeutic progress, which is rewarding and motivating for therapists and clients alike. In addition, it is suggested that, by adopting a more thoughtful approach in advance of embarking on goal planning or direct intervention, workload is lessened rather than increased.

This approach may mean therapists having to develop a wider knowledge base, having to renegotiate relationships or information flow with colleagues, or having to rethink the style of service delivery. But overall, the application of the principles that underpin this approach should result in more responsive, efficient and effective service provision.

This chapter, then, outlines the importance of including consideration of a particular set of potential influencing factors, described as the impact of the traumatic event and the influence of life context, when addressing the optimal physiotherapeutic contribution within a programme of rehabilitation after traumatic brain injury (TBI). In addition, it stresses the need to consider these factors as they apply to friends and family as well as to the injured individual. The particular relevance of this approach to TBI rehabilitation, and the need for such width of knowledge, is explored, and examples of both the positive effects of adopting the proposed approach and the negative consequences of failing to do so are given.

THE IMPACT OF THE TRAUMATIC EVENT

From the moment a TBI occurs that is serious enough for medical advice to be sought, a series of events and experiences ensue that impact on the person who sustains the injury and on those who are closest to them. When an individual who has sustained a TBI first presents for medical evaluation, and in severe injuries for some considerable time during the life preservation period, the focus of the medical team is by necessity on body systems and pathological signs and symptoms. This period progresses, in the main, independently of any influence external to the medical process. Many medical management decisions are made under pressure of time and, except for the necessary consents for surgical intervention, there is rarely reference to anything outside the medical process.

In effect, the responsibility for making decisions transfers to the medical team and this puts them in control. It is hard to imagine many other circumstances where such a spontaneous transfer of responsibility takes place, where an individual loses control, sometimes to the extent of being reliant on a machine for life giving breath.

There is no question that it is appropriate for control to transfer to those who have the knowledge to make the necessary decisions and the skills to deliver the necessary care. It is essential, however, that healthcare practitioners do not assume control beyond what is necessary and endeavour to share decision-making responsibilities when appropriate.

From the point of injury and throughout the process of recovery and rehabilitation, the experience of the injured person and the experience of those who are close to them will be different. However, one of the primary components of the professional relationship between service providers and service users in the aftermath of TBI is the process by which the maximal amount of control and responsibility is returned to the injured individual or to their support network.

THE EXPERIENCE OF FRIENDS AND FAMILIES

Much of this book has a strong focus on the injured individual, how they present to rehabilitation services and to individual therapists. Presumably, therapists who read this book are concerned with how they might intervene physically to improve individuals' physical abilities and functional outcome. However, as will become increasingly apparent throughout the text of this book, the effects of TBI are rarely transient: they are often lifelong and, as such, impact on whole families (Brooks & McKinlay 1983, Brooks et al 1987, Romano 1974, Rosenbaum & Najenson 1976). Therapists need to work with friends and families as well as injured individuals and, to do so effectively, they need to understand the families' experiences.

To highlight the kinds of issue that friends and family have to deal with, some illustrative examples from clinical experience are given below. Not all of the examples apply to everyone and the content is not fully inclusive. The examples do, however, give some indication of the magnitude of emotional and practical issues that may be encountered by family members, and they have obvious implications for service providers. Further personal descriptions and retrospective accounts have been published and make informative reading (Beaver 1991, Hardgrove 1991, Kramer 1991, Rees 1988).

Attempts have also been made to conceptualize the carers' experience (Douglas 1990, Hopewell et al 1989, Talbott 1989, Williams 1991) in order to describe common responses and progressions. Douglas (1990) offers a five-stage model, with subtext for each of the stages (Fig. 3.1). In referring to this work, Ponsford (1995) makes the important observation that the sequence and rate of progression through these stages will not be the same for every family and that not all families will pass through all stages. I would also add that it is necessary to consider that individual members of the same family may also vary in their responses, which can make it difficult for them to support one another and may give a poor impression of the family to professionals and other outsiders. With these provisos, Douglas's model is a useful structural guide and I will refer to her categories within case examples.

The acute phase

Hospitals are alien environments for the majority of the general population. They have their own culture, vocabulary, and policies and procedures that are adopted as routine by employees. Although many of the routines and regulations are developed from a sound medical or organizational

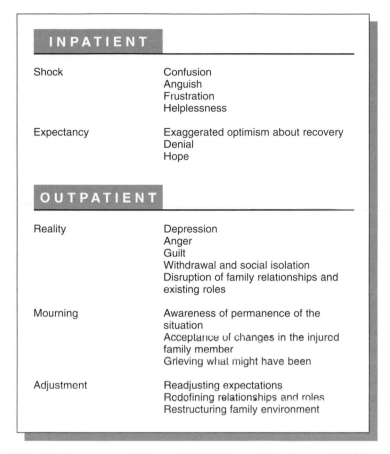

Figure 3.1   Family response to traumatic brain injury: a five-stage model. From Douglas (1990)

basis, they can appear unnecessary or even divisive to friends and family who want to be close to their loved one. For example, restrictions on timing of visits or on numbers of visitors may be necessary for the care of the individual or the efficiency of the wider ward. From the relatives' point of view, however, this may be viewed as unnecessary bureaucracy or a lack of acknowledgement of their needs.

At the same time as much of the intensive medical intervention is taking place, friends and relatives are experiencing a variety of destabilizing emotional processes. There is an initial period of *shock*, which may manifest itself in a number of ways. Some individuals appear unreasonably calm, others may be forgetful or confused in other ways.

As well as the unfamiliarity of the hospital environment, there are many other unknowns to deal with. First, what will the outcome be? Will their loved one survive? If they do, what lasting effect might the injuries have?

Relatives will have been told that damage to the brain has occurred, but that the extent of the damage and the long-term effects cannot be predicted accurately. They will have been told that the first few days are crucial and maybe that the medical team has done all that is possible and now everyone has simply to wait and see. People deal with the uncertainties of this situation in different ways.

Many relatives describe their approach in retrospect as simply preparing themselves for the worst, bracing themselves for the loss that they feel may be imminent. Some describe having experienced feelings of guilt when their loved one did survive because they felt that, by preparing for the worst, they had given up on them. Some describe experiencing shear elation when their loved one opened their eyes or showed some other sign of life activity, and a significant number say that at the same point they believed that everything would be all right, no matter what they may have been told by the professionals.

When discussing this period in retrospect it is not uncommon for carers to describe their reasoning at this time in a similar way to these sentiments expressed by one mother:

Well, the doctors said that there was a 90% chance that David wouldn't survive and he did, so, they got that wrong and I was determined to prove that they were wrong when they said that he would never walk again.

David's mother could be characterized as being in the stage of expectancy, optimistic about recovery and denying the possibility that medical advice could be correct.

This apparently adversarial attitude is commonly observed in carers (McLaughlin & Carey 1993), some from very early on. For example, another parent described uncontainable anger when the neurosurgeon who assessed his son told him that there was no surgical operation that could help and that the prognosis was very poor. He said:

I felt they had just discarded Peter, that they were making no effort and I couldn't just sit there by his bed like my wife did. I was angry with her too, just sitting accepting it all, I wanted somebody to do something, you know, run around like they do on the telly. It seemed like everyone was so laid back, moving around almost in slow motion when they should have been doing something to make him better.

Peter's parents clearly demonstrated a different response to the same circumstances and information, and his father was able to acknowledge (months later) how he blamed his wife for not responding in the same way that he did. At the time of his conversation with me, which had developed from an apparently unconnected discussion (of transport issues), Peter's father had not been able to tell his wife about his feelings.

Some months later, Peter's mother indicated that they had discussed some of these issues and that she had also been angry during the acute period because Peter's father would not sit with him. She had felt that close family members should be at Peter's bedside in case he should wake up and had felt burdened by the whole of this responsibility falling to her.

From the standpoint of an outside observer, this early experience had influenced their ongoing roles, with mother continuing to be the direct caregiver and father being the practical organizer. However, although this pattern could be seen, and neither was happy with the imbalance in their role, change was achieved only slowly and partially because of issues like Peter's mother feeling that the discussion of change indicated a criticism of her performance as caregiver.

Other carers describe a similar sense of helplessness, of not having anything to offer or of being unable to find anyway to help while 'these complete strangers are doing it all'. Sometimes carers have been confused by inconsistencies in practice on the ward, for example having a varying level of involvement depending on the approach of the senior nurse on duty.

Of course, families bring with them to the traumatic experience their positive and their negative attributes. We have only to think about our own families and circle of friends to recognize the type of strained relationships or unfinished business that would be around between the major players if we were the person who had sustained the injury. Dominant family members can take over, rationing access to others and preventing them from contributing to care. Without a direct care role, friends and family members tend to drift away leaving, in the end, the burden of care with the dominant member.

As a substantial amount of evidence begins to emerge that family coping in the long term is linked with the notion and practicalities of having a well functioning family and extended support network (Douglas 1996, Perlesz et al 1996), it would seem important not to allow such divisions to occur. Hospital systems can contribute to painful exclusions, for example by automatically affording parents the role of next of kin without due consideration of a cohabiting partner. This sort of disenfranchisement has occurred, in my experience, for non-married partners in heterosexual and homosexual relationships, and has resulted in significant ongoing difficulties through the rehabilitation and adjustment phase.

In the same way as this chapter aims to place the injured individual within the context of the wider family system, it also aims to promote recognition that carers themselves have lives and responsibilities beyond the hospital ward. In the immediate acute period through the phases of shock and expectancy and into the dawning of reality, carers' lives are often put on hold, impacting on children, parents, work, and so on. For carers, achieving a healthy balance between all these responsibilities, and taking time to meet their own needs, is rarely possible without external support and assistance, and yet it is still a common experience for carers not only to be unsupported but often to be in a position of fighting for services appropriate to their loved one's needs.

Preparing for hospital discharge

From the time of regaining consciousness or recovery from surgical intervention, the aim of achieving discharge to home becomes a major focus for families and professionals alike. It is impossible to detail all the probable issues to be dealt with during this period, and the length of the subacute period will vary enormously for each individual.

It has been noted by a number of authors, however, that this is commonly a time of great expectation and conversely a time when it is difficult for carers to accept that existing deficits will be other than transient (Hopewell et al 1989, Oddy 1995, Rosenthal 1989). There is relief that life has been preserved, often in the face of the grim predictions of medical personnel. Where the injured individual demonstrates agitation, confusion or other behavioural disturbance in the early subacute period, relatives and friends may be embarrassed and often bewildered as to why someone who essentially looks to be the same person is behaving in such an atypical manner.

The presence of physical deficits provides a tangible focus for the need for intervention or continued hospital stay. However, the more abstract notions of potential cognitive deficits are much more difficult to comprehend and, indeed, are often attributed to the hospital environment or even to failures in care. An example of the difficulty of this kind of situation from my own experience is given in Case example 3.1.

It is worth noting that where the TBI does not result in an extended period of intensive care, or when the initial deficits do not include major physical dysfunction or obvious gross cognitive difficulties, carers often find themselves at home with the injured individual in a matter of hours or within a few days. These carers generally do not have access to explanation or information about what to expect; indeed, they are likely to have been told that full recovery is to be anticipated, and may not interpret any continuing complaints as being related to the original injury. While many individuals will recover from such a mild or moderate injury in days, weeks or a few months, there is a small minority who continue to experience difficulties, which may include physical symptoms such as dizziness, visual disturbance or headache.

The early period at home

Depending on a variety of factors, such as the severity and type of the ongoing deficits, the length of inpatient stay and their progress towards understanding the reality of the situation, families' experiences of the

---

Case example 3.1   Terry

In addition to a TBI, Terry also sustained lower limb fractures. On emergence from coma he was bed/chairbound and clearly in need of continuing care. His wife and family accepted the need for him to be transferred to a rehabilitative facility. However, in the space of less than 2 weeks, he could transfer and walk a few steps with the aid of two crutches.

At the same time he started exhibiting intolerant, agitated and sometimes tearful behaviour, especially when family members were present. Terry had a language deficit somewhat akin to the fluent dysphasia more commonly associated with stroke. His agitation and stream of confused expressive output was interpreted by his family as discontentment with the hospital regime, and they responded to his repetitive 'demands for home' by promoting an almost immediate discharge, against the wishes of the inpatient rehabilitation team.

Terry's local community disability service was designed on a client empowerment basis, with the laudable intention of allowing individuals to choose to be supported in their own home if they were medically stable and wished to be at home. The problem here was that this process of self-determination was not balanced by any consideration of whether Terry was in position to express informed consent or what the impact on the family of sustaining the home discharge would be. Thus, the physical adaptations were promptly provided to facilitate discharge home and he was referred to the specialist outpatient service where I worked.

Instead of the anticipated calm as a result of his return home to familiar circumstances and attentive care, his demanding behaviour escalated. Initially he was similarly agitated, and subsequently a pattern of behaviour emerged of alternating withdrawal and explosive outbursts. Terry's wife, having insisted on her husband's discharge, felt that she would need to cope and, even when given openings by myself and colleagues to say otherwise, insisted for almost a year afterwards that everything at home was OK. She was loyal and uncritical of her husband, highlighting only minimal deficits during the initial outpatient assessment process.

One year later she was able to admit that all was not well and the details of her husband's demanding and often frightening behaviour began to emerge. However, this was not before their grown-up daughter, who previously had happily cohabited with her parents in the family home, had opted to move out. Subsequent to that move she too began to open up, describing the 'tyranny' of her father and making it clear that she felt her mother should leave as well.

It was established several months into his outpatient programme that Terry, in retrospect, had no personal recall of his time in the inpatient rehabilitation facility. This is despite the fact that for many months he used a repetitive phrase (one of many) within conversation that he did not like the [city name] in which the facility was housed. This was taken by the family to mean the facility itself, but Terry's confusion or limited reasoning was also evident in that this soon developed into an absolute ban on travel to anywhere in the city of the same name. Given that our specialist outpatient facility is also in the same city, there had to be a considerable amount of liaison with locally based therapists who, having gained Terry's confidence, eventually persuaded him to attend for outpatient assessment.

---

early days at home can be quite varied. Families usually experience what has often been described as a honeymoon period, being in their own safe environment and, on the face of it, re-establishing the normal family unit.

However, as the optimism and hope of *expectancy* are challenged by the daily experiences of a changed reality, many carers experience increasing levels of distress. Whereas distress, depression and anxiety in primary carers have been found by some authors to diminish from initial high levels over the hospital period (Novack et al 1991, Oddy et al 1978), there is also evidence to suggest that, for some, these factors begin to rise again after discharge home (Brooks & McKinlay 1983, Livingston et al 1985, McKinlay et al 1981).

These effects are not restricted to the carers of persons sustaining severe head injury. In a survey of consecutive attendees over a 3-month period recorded as sustaining a TBI at accident and emergency facilities in Sheffield, UK, with follow-up interview at 6 months' postinjury, one third of the relatives interviewed were found to have significantly high levels of psychological distress (Telford & Wright 1992). The full sample had an incidence of minor injury (Glasgow Coma Score 13–14) of 85% and the interview sample 90%.

At 2.5 years an attempt was made to follow up the relatives of 24 of those with loss of consciousness of less than 15 min, who had been interviewed at 6 months; this proved difficult. Thirteen declined to be interviewed, three families were untraceable and there had been one death. However, although scores on the General Health Questionnaire (Goldberg & Williams 1988) of the eight interviewed were not now significantly different from those of a control group, a significant difference remained with regard to the Impact of Event Scale (Horowitz et al 1979).

The authors correctly advise caution in the interpretation of these findings but also suggest that a larger-scale examination of the impact of a minor TBI on relatives is needed (Telford & Wright 1996).

A tangible example from my own experience of the effect of the length of time at home following discharge from inpatient care is the level of difficulties reported by carers as part of the initial outpatient assessment. Although not set up as a formal comparative study, the response rate of our outpatient service has varied over the years. At times when there has been no waiting list for assessment and clients have come for assessment immediately, or sometimes even before hospital discharge, the reported levels of current difficulties have been low. When there has been a moderate wait of, say, less than 2 months, concrete functional examples of difficulties begin to be more frequently reported. And when the waiting period has been longer, especially where there has been no interim support, the personal distress of the carer is often very tangible, leading to lengthy and emotional carer interviews.

Adjusting to the new situation

How families move from beginning to be aware of some permanence in the changed situation through the period described by Douglas (1990) as *mourning* to some level of adjustment is a complex and individual process.

Much of the research reported to date has been concerned with identifying and documenting the painful process and trying to establish what factors have a direct bearing on relatives' distress. Whereas in the early days of recovery subjective burden appears to be linked to providing physical care (Marsh et al 1996), there is much evidence to link the social and functional effects of cognitive and behavioural deficits to continuing levels of subjective burden (Brooks & McKinlay 1983, Brooks et al 1987, Cavallo et al 1992, Douglas 1996, Frosch et al 1997, Gleckman & Brill 1995, Junque et al 1997, Leaf 1993, Leatham et al 1996, Oddy 1995, Rosenbaum & Najenson 1976). As the impact of TBI on the family can no longer be in doubt, research now has begun to focus on how the effect can be minimized and how family coping and adjustment may be facilitated.

It is not strictly accurate to make comparisons across published studies, as samples are not equivalent. There are some points of interest worth high-lighting, however, which can help inform service planning and identify areas requiring further formal research.

The early studies, published in the 1970s and 1980s, are based mainly on populations that had no access to any form of coordinated post-acute rehabilitation and had limited postdischarge support. Not surprisingly, they reported higher levels of subjective burden than studies linked with intervention programmes.

While a number of studies are skewed towards the early recovery phase and do not track carers further down the line, some more recent community-based studies are emerging. For example, Douglas (1996) confirmed the presence of continuing family distress in a severely injured population up to 10 years postinjury, and also identified the adequacy of carers' social support as a significant indicator of good family functioning even in the presence of cognitive and behavioural factors that carers acknowledged having difficulty dealing with.

Perlesz (1996), in a study looking at primary, secondary and tertiary carers, identified unexpected levels of distress in tertiary carers, for example siblings with little responsibility for caring for the injured family member. Perlesz is keen to move some of the focus for further research towards looking at those families that do adjust and do cope, so that service providers may understand the salient factors for positive outcome.

THE EXPERIENCE OF THE INDIVIDUAL

The experience of injured individuals throughout the whole process is different to that of their friends and families. If we consider the medical management and recovery process outlined in Chapter 2, it is possible to begin to envisage a typical progression through a number of key stages that will have a direct impact on the injured individual's perspective.

The acute phase

During the primary acute phase, many injured individuals have a period of spontaneous or medically induced coma (see Ch. 2). This time, which may span several weeks or even months, is forever lost to them, a period that is missing from their lives. Similarly, any period of transient confusion – of post-traumatic amnesia – will also be missing from their recall.

Unlike those who watch and hope for their recovery, the injured person has no concept of the life and death situation that they may be in and, as they emerge into a more oriented state of being, they may easily fail to appreciate how serious their predicament has been. When they do start to connect with their environment, their world is not what they expect to find.

When someone has been unconscious as a result of TBI, they do not usually move straight from the unconscious state to one of clarity. There is often a period of fluctuating awareness, presumably giving them a series of disjointed snapshots of an unfamiliar world as they alternately wake and sleep and spend time in disorienting periods of waking confusion. This period may be further complicated by communication difficulties, of being unable to express anxieties or ask questions, or in failing to make sense of what is being said. It is hardly surprising that agitation and disruptive or other atypical behaviours are prominent features at this time.

It has already been noted that this is often a distressing time for carers, and it is my experience that this is also the case for the injured person, possibly more in retrospect than at the time of occurrence.

Many of my clients have confided a wide range of negative feelings in relation to their knowledge of their behaviour during this period. Some are simply embarrassed or mildly confused by what they have been told and can be reassured by explanations of the period of fluctuating consciousness and one or two examples of other people's abnormal behaviours. Others have found the whole idea that other people know more about what happened to them and what they were doing for a period of their lives a difficult concept to deal with. This has been particularly the case when families have continued to make reference to the atypical behaviours, especially in insensitive ways, for example at family gatherings.

Preparing for discharge

The drive to return home from hospital is strong and appears to be the primary concern of many individuals from the early subacute stage. Professionals working in the field of TBI can produce legions of anecdotal reports of successful and failed 'escape' attempts by those who do not, or cannot, accept the need to remain in hospital. As has been highlighted by the case example of Terry, barriers to coping at home are often seen as primarily physical and when there are no such barriers, or the possibility of them being overcome is introduced, it is often difficult to come up with a rationale for continued inpatient treatment that the client will find accept-able. This problem of limited self-awareness of deficits other than physical dysfunction within routine care tasks is well recognized in the literature (Fleming et al 1996, Prigatano & Altman 1990, Prigatano & Fordyce 1986).

The hospital environment is alien and detached from the injured per-son's 'normal' life. Although the incidence of memory dysfunction after TBI is significant, this rarely involves those aspects of memory concerned with past life. Even when there is partial loss of recall, this usually affects the immediate preinjury period (retrograde amnesia), and the injured per-son still has an impression of their past life, their main life roles and leisure pursuits.

In Chapter 2, the TBI population was described as typically young, in the majority male, and in many cases to have sustained the injuries during what may be termed risk-taking activities. It has also been noted that a sig-nificant subsection of the TBI population comes from backgrounds where, for example, they may have experienced an unsatisfactory education, been unemployed at the time of injury or, if employed, were in a low-paid job (Rimel et al 1990).

Additional consideration has to be given to the significant number who may have misused drugs or alcohol or have a history of a previous TBI, with obvious or latent effect on their life. When the inpatient environment is far removed from the preinjury lifestyle recalled by the injured person, they might have difficulty accepting guidance or advice from the associated professional staff.

In addition, as many professionals are concerned with basing interven-tions on objective assessments, the delay in actioning a meaningful pro-gramme and the process of formal assessment itself may serve to confirm the feeling of irrelevance. The general population equates being in hospi-tal with being ill and, even when they have some premorbid understand-ing of the existence of rehabilitation, this is commonly regarded as relating to physical ability. If the injured individual feels neither ill nor unable to cope from a physical point of view, they reasonably expect to be at home.

Professionals as yet do not approach the issue of discrepancy between their own interpretation of the probable impact of apparent impairment and that of the injured person from a common standpoint. The knowledge base within and across disciplines is inconsistent and there is much still to be learned. From a pragmatic point of view, however, it seems undeniable that people cannot be expected to understand the consequences or impact of deficits they are unaware of, and this applies to all people, whether lay or professional.

It is to be hoped that future research will result in clearer guidelines for less experienced professionals in relation to the process of adjustment.

Until then, professionals can proceed on the basis of at least understanding that 'insight' is not a quality possessed or not possessed by clients or carers, but a result of a learning process that cannot be achieved without the reception of adequate information or appropriate experience. The quantity of information that is given, how it is given and how learning experiences may be structured are matters for careful team discussion. In addition, it is essential that the demands made on the individual run at a parallel level to the stage of understanding.

It is also important to recognize that, in the same way as they have limited awareness of the deficits and their potential functional impact, the injured person is unlikely to be aware of the potential impact of their changed status on those who care for them. And, although the carers may think about their own ability to manage any physical difficulties in the short term, they are unlikely to anticipate the effects of these demands if they continue over time, or the special pressures of dealing with effects of cognitive deficits on themselves and the wider family. There is, therefore, a role for professionals to aid balanced decision making in terms of discharge timing and process, and to lobby strongly for appropriate support from care organizations and from the potential wide support network of family and friends.

Tyerman (1991) advocates a counselling approach, which runs parallel to the rest of the rehabilitation process, to address many of these interlinked issues. Highlighting the complex set of adjustments required of the injured person and of their family, he has delineated a process of four phases:

- Acute care
- Rehabilitation
- Resettlement
- Long-term adjustment.

Tyerman does not recommend a psychotherapeutic approach within the first three phases, rather the development of a relationship of trust for giving information and repeated explanations in a sensitive way and becoming more detailed as recovery progresses. Within this relationship there is opportunity to raise concerns about the likely course and extent of recovery to enable an increased understanding of what has happened and what might be anticipated. Tyerman suggests that regular counselling can play a crucial role in the monitoring and review of treatment goals and, as such, it may usefully be carried out by an appointed key worker, who can be from any of the rehabilitation professions.

What he describes is essentially a process whereby education, support and advice are linked with the practical rehabilitation process so that both parties can make use of tangible examples or action changes in the programme in response to the ongoing discussion. Although Tyerman acknowledges that many individuals will experience periods of low mood, particularly as they become more aware of the impact of their impairments, he asserts that, with the backup of a clinical neuropsychologist, much of the *routine* counselling work in this regard can be carried out by other team members in the course of their work. The more complex cases can then be addressed directly by the psychologist.

Beyond the routine rehabilitation counselling, which Tyerman (1991, p. 124) describes as 'providing information and explanation, promoting insight and realistic expectations and planning appropriately for re-settlement', the final stage is then 'to assist people to re-appraise their new situation and achieve the difficult balance whereby they accommodate the consequences of their injury without also being governed by them'. When there is difficulty with the latter stage, he suggests it is appropriate to adopt a more psychotherapeutic approach, with adequate compensation for cognitive limitations. Some of the potential difficulties that may be anticipated during the *resettlement* and *long-term adjustment* phases are discussed below.

Dealing with the real world

After discharge from inpatient care there is great variety in the ways in which injured individuals begin to re-engage with their previous environment and life habits. Much is dependent upon the level at which they are functioning and how far removed they are from attempting to return to their previous primary activity, such as work, home management or study.

Other personal factors have an impact, for example whether they are able to return to their own home or whether they require others to contribute to their care in what they may regard as an intrusive way. Another major factor is whether or not there is continued planned contact with rehabilitation services and, when there is, whether those services are perceived as appropriate.

It would be inappropriate to imply that every person who returns home during the process of recovery following TBI has the same experience. It is also of interest to note that, while most of the resources associated with medical, rehabilitative and social care are undoubtedly focused on the person who has sustained the injury, there is, in contrast to the research work relating to families, little attention given in the literature to attempts to define the stages of a recovery–adjustment process for injured individuals. However, it is clear that where recovery is not to the extent that allows immediate return to all preinjury activities, each individual will be faced with the need to adjust to changed circumstances. This process may be traumatic and is sometimes incomplete.

Adjustment to enforced change is always difficult and for the injured person with impaired cognitive abilities there are additional complexities.

In addition, the characteristics of the population, for example the predominance of the young, the newly married, the presence of children or a lack of preinjury stability in lifestyle, add complicating factors which conspire to limit the effects of efforts made by the individual and professionals alike. Where professionals are unaware of these issues, or when that awareness is not translated into service provision or design, the confusion of the individual at this time can be interpreted as a lack of motivation or a straightforward inability to progress.

Also, with the increasing emphasis on goal-directed therapy, the inability of the individual to identify goals or their apparent failure to work toward the goals identified for them by the professionals may again result in the withdrawal of services. Where services are organized in a way that allows one bite of the cherry fairly early on in the recovery period, an inability to engage the individual at this time may well mean the end of rehabilitation before it has in fact begun.

IMPLICATIONS FOR SERVICE PROVIDERS

There are a few principles for service providers implied by the preceding discussion. More detailed suggestions concerning comprehensive service design are examined in Chapter 10.

INFORMATION AND SUPPORT

Families and others affected by the trauma of the injury and the period of acute medical management, need access to accurate information. The information needs to be presented in a format that allows the development of a true understanding of its content. This may mean providing the information in a variety of formats or giving the same information on repeated occasions. It certainly means that all professionals approached should be able to give the same appropriate information or to refer the questioner to a resource where that information will be available. Families need to be able to question, if they do not recall, do not understand or do not want to believe the information they have been given. Clinical experience is that they will feel more able to ask questions if they perceive they are supported.

In Sheffield, as part of a UK Department of Health Initiative, we established a Specialist Head Injury Social Work Team, which had the aim of providing immediate and ongoing support for carers from day 1 if they wished, and throughout the period of contact with the rehabilitation services. In practice this meant making an initial contact within the first few days, giving a contact number and being as active a supporter as relevant to each particular family unit. Families and individual members used this service in a variety of ways, some early on, some only at points of service change, some only with regard to practical issues, and others much later in the process when the injured person had returned home.

For a variety of organizational and resource reasons, the working pattern of this small two-person team was not consistently sustained after the initial 2-year period and at the time of writing is not able to work into the acute stage. However, subjective reports gathered by interviewers independent of the service as part of the evaluation revealed that this aspect of the service was highly valued by all carers. In addition, therapists and social work staff who had been involved in the service before this development noted that there was a qualitative difference in carers' approach and attitude at the beginning of the outpatient stage.

A retrospective review of activity also revealed a concurrent increase in the numbers of active cases being dealt with by the outpatient team, which could not be accounted for by increased therapeutic resources. This appeared to validate the subjective feeling that therapeutic goals were easier to progress because family crises and unexpected complicating developments were less frequent.

ONGOING NEEDS OF CARERS

Beyond the obvious need for good-quality information and support in the acute period, service provision needs to recognize the specific needs of carers throughout the rehabilitation period. In pragmatic terms, rehabilitation goals are extremely difficult to achieve in the presence of family distress, and meaningful rehabilitation goals are not easy to negotiate with families who have become and remain angry.

Even when early service provision has been adequate and when carers do not feel critical, they still have much to deal with in recognizing the permanence of the changes that face them and in coming to terms with the effects of those changes. Many caregivers exhaust their personal resources over the first year or so and, without encouragement to pace their involvement, become unable to contribute constructively to the ongoing rehabilitation programmes.

For some, effective provision may mean advice and guidance that allows them to return to their own employment, breaking the cycle of care and introducing some balance in their lives. For others, it may mean the practical provision of substitute carers or escorts for children, for example to maintain their leisure pursuits. In specific cases it may be education with regard to the principles and practice of behavioural management, or help to establish a flexible planning and organization regime.

The point is that assessment of needs should take place in respect of the immediate family unit and even if resources will not run to direct provision then at least we should know not to make additional demands on an already stressed system.

The effects of discharge from the rehabilitation system on carers should not be underestimated. It is sometimes only after the structure and regular contact are removed that some individuals begin to recognize the permanence and/or severity of their situation. I have been surprised by a number of people who had appeared to be coping well with their situation and who had taken an active part in the discussions about rehabilitation goals and the decision regarding discharge, but who later reported being distraught when the discharge actually occurred.

One articulate mother described fluctuating between two extremes on the day of the family review meeting where discharge was being confirmed. Her son had not attended the outpatient centre for almost 6 months and it had been agreed and clearly documented at a previous meeting that discharge would occur if the unsupported review period went smoothly. She said that she had come with the intention of thanking all the staff for their assistance and support and proudly to report on how well the review period had gone. But, as she entered the centre, she became suddenly aware of the finality of the event and was overcome by a feeling of panic. She did deliver her thanks and she, her husband and her son did report their previous 6 months in largely positive terms. She showed no outward signs of panic. However, she phoned the centre on some pretence less than a week later and reiterated her thanks during the conversation as she was sure she had failed to do so during the visit. Although she had appeared relaxed and in full control during the meeting, she had no clear recall of the content afterwards, only that she had been overcome by an emotional response and presumed that she had failed to contribute.

In another instance a woman whose husband had sustained a serious TBI denied any problems throughout the rehabilitation programme. In fact, the therapists involved in this case had been very concerned about the situation at home but had not been able to engage the family in either the planning or delivery of the programme. And, while some progress was achieved within therapy sessions, only a small degree of change was achieved at home. This was despite developing a variety of ideas and attempting a number of approaches to aid discussion. The therapists were at first surprised that the woman kept the appointment as she had cancelled others at the last minute and had even not been at home on occasion when visits had been arranged. She sat through the meeting acknowledging a number of issues as they were discussed and towards the end of the meeting simply began to cry. Up until that point she had presented as coping practically and resenting attempts at contact. Fortunately, although her husband was discharged from our service it was possible to identify local psychological help for her. It is of note that, although it had previously proved impossible for her to acknowledge need or accept assistance, at the point of discharge when the reality seemed to suddenly hit her, her need was immediate.

When structured rehabilitation comes to an end, the majority of care, in its widest sense, returns to the family. If support networks have survived, the burden can be shared either directly or indirectly. However, even when much of the routine care is absorbed by these primary caregivers and their support network, there is still need for access to specialist advice to deal with unusual occurrences or to assist at times when other demands on families reduce their ability to cope. Moreover, for some people this need for knowledgeable backup, and sometimes practical respite, continues for the rest of the injured person's life.

COLLABORATION AND CONSISTENCY

Achieving consistency of approach and clarity in giving information requires appropriate service planning and maintenance. Confusion and dissatisfaction can be minimized by collaborative working between the professionals, but collaboration needs to be facilitated by the style of service provision.

Interdisciplinary team working in the field of TBI has been highlighted in the literature as the ideal for almost two decades. Seamless services and pathways of care are suggested to facilitate progress and to remove some of the uncertainty from an already traumatic process. However, with competing demands and financial constraints, these intentions, even when established in practice, have proven difficult to maintain.

There is a basic knowledge issue at the generic level, which is common to most health professions. Therapists, medical staff, nurses, health policy makers and purchasers of healthcare do not, on the whole, receive a vast amount of education relating to the potential long-term effects of TBI or of the impact on the health and well-being of families. TBI provision is often catered for as an add-on to other areas of responsibility and, whether this is at planning, purchasing or service delivery level, it often means learning on the job. The healthcare workforce is fluid and mobile, and existing patterns of career progression, especially for therapists, do not support advanced clinical practice. It is unusual for the learning period to be followed by any length of informed activity and it is more common that, when experienced personnel leave to progress in their career, they are replaced by someone who is back at the beginning of the learning curve.

It is only when health and social care provision and the costs and benefits to the exchequer are considered as a whole that the financial cost of not providing meaningful rehabilitation and support services is identified. And it is only when therapists and other health professionals think longitudinally and act collaboratively that the potentially negative or positive impact of their contribution can be fully appreciated. This means thinking beyond the contribution of their discipline within their service and beyond their service to consider how they fit into the wider picture.

THE INFLUENCE OF LIFE CONTEXT

As well as being aware of the impact of the spiral of events that follows the initial trauma, therapists need also to understand the importance of acknowledging the influence of life context during assessment, goal planning and intervention design. The practicalities of information gathering, discussion and negotiation of intervention goals and the use of accumulated knowledge to aid effective programme design are all covered in detail in later chapters.

What is highlighted here is, first, what is meant by life context and, second, why such a focus is considered necessary. In addition we will look, in practical terms, at individual and familial characteristics that may have implications for the style and content of assessment and intervention. The aim is twofold: to raise awareness of the need to look towards real life in rehabilitation planning and to inform therapists so that they may set appropriate targets and make reasonable demands. Discussion will include examples of barriers to success as a result of failing to consider life context. In contrast, the potential for improving outcome by the creative use of the accumulated knowledge will also be described briefly.

WHAT IS MEANT BY LIFE CONTEXT?

Life context refers to the individual, their relationships and lifestyle before the injury and since the injury has occurred. For ease of discussion, the relevant factors are outlined with reference to three areas. The first relates to the individual, the second to the family unit, and the third to the wider culture and community within which the first two operate.

The individual

The potential global effects of TBI on an individual's brain, and therefore on their functional ability, have been described in the previous chapter. We have already seen that, in addition to the more obvious immediate effects on conscious level and physical functioning, many people who sustain a TBI also experience subtle or substantial changes in cognitive ability and in their behavioural presentation. However, when someone who has sustained a TBI is referred to a physiotherapist, especially in the hospital environment, it is easy for the physiotherapist simply to focus on the presenting sensorimotor problems, designing management and intervention strategies to tackle the immediate physical findings.

It is, of course, highly appropriate for the physiotherapist, as a specialist in the analysis of movement and physical methods of remediation, to assess and treat sensorimotor dysfunction. However, this assessment and treatment does not take place in a vacuum. Physiotherapists need to understand the whole dynamic within which they operate so that they may become effective specialist practitioners within the multiprofessional team. If the outcome of their intervention is to be meaningful to the injured person, the process of assessment, goal setting, and choice and application of intervention strategy should reflect wider considerations, such as the person's individuality and preinjury lifestyle.

What is meant by individuality?

The brain, more than any other part of us, defines our individuality. It is the repository of our particular and unique memories, the controller of our defining skills and abilities, the moderator of our characteristic moods and feelings, the facilitator of our interactions with our environment and our communications with our fellow human beings. (Rose & Johnson 1996, p. 1)

If we accept that many of our clients will have diffuse brain injury then this quote highlights the scope of disturbance that they may experience.

It is beyond the remit of this book to examine in any detail concepts of individuality or models of behaviour. However, there is no question that each one of us has a sense of our own identity and that our identity is placed within a particular cultural context. It is not necessarily something that we consciously attend to or think about, but in normal circumstances our process of development through childhood, adolescence and into adulthood combines our basic personal characteristics with our life experiences. By way of this process we develop behavioural characteristics, a particular outlook on life and, to a lesser or greater extent, an anticipation of what we might expect to do or achieve in the future.

It is important to recognize that, at the point of sustaining injury, each individual is somewhere along this developmental continuum and has a view of themselves and their world that is individual to them. And, if the purpose of the rehabilitation process is to promote a meaningful functional outcome, it is important to gain some understanding of where the individual is on the developmental continuum and whether or not, for example, they hold particular life views or have specific life goals.

Practical applications of knowledge of the individual

The importance of therapists and others holding appropriate knowledge in the acute stage is exemplified by considering the likelihood of the presence of altered consciousness, confusion or agitation. Appropriate reassurance can be given or, if necessary, reorientation to reality in the presence of confabulation.

It is also important to gain an understanding of the roles and responsibilities held by the injured person and to apply that knowledge in the approach to intervention. Are they a parent, a child living at home, a young adult living away from home, a businessperson, a rally driver?

Some of this information may be used to help the therapist suggest functional goals to gain motivation or to promote attention to a task. In other circumstances, background information can be used to inform all team members' responses to inquiries relating to potential recovery and likely functional outcome. It is essential to ensure that these responses are well founded and consistent, and that they do not inflate expectations or cause undue pessimism.

Beyond the acute period, knowledge of preinjury life goals and plans are again essential to help anticipate the individual's thoughts in relation to their predicament. We as healthcare professionals may see the individual as a person who has sustained a TBI, but they will see themselves as a distinct individual and as someone who has one or more specific roles within their own family system, for example student, mother, family wage earner, family pacifier, and so on.

As can be seen in relating the potential deficits to the role of the brain in defining individuality, while major disruptions in function are present the injured person may have difficulty linking knowledge of their premorbid lifestyle with rehabilitation goals. They might have a clear memory of their role in life or their preferred activities before their injury, and their stated intent may be to return to that role and those activities; however, they are unlikely to be able to identify a clear route towards those end goals.

Knowledge of their premorbid lifestyle can help therapists to facilitate the injured person in the identification of short- and medium-term goals with overt links to possible long-term goals that will feel appropriate. This knowledge can be used repeatedly throughout the rehabilitation process and, although it may be impossible to work towards or achieve a full set of preinjury goals or aspirations, it is usually possible to embrace some aspects of these goals and at least to work within the spirit of the previous intent until specific long-term goals can be identified and appropriate adjustments encouraged.

I should stress that I am not recommending that every goal identified by the injured person should be taken on board, no matter how outlandish or unrealistic it may be. Equally, I am not implying that everyone who has sustained a TBI is likely to return to all their preinjury activities. What I am saying is that rehabilitation goals will be achieved more easily if a tangible link is made between the therapeutic activity and real life aspirations.

In TBI rehabilitation, given the length of the potential rehabilitation period and the likelihood of deficits affecting understanding, reasoning and other cognitive processes, limiting the patient's ability to make their own links, the process of overtly linking therapeutic activities to real life aspirations is valuable on many levels. Also, even when the ultimate outcome may be less than was originally hoped for, it will not be seen as being because of lack of focus on issues relevant to the client.

The family or primary support network

In the same way as it is important to recognize the individuality of injured persons, it is equally important to understand the special characteristics of the family. The family system or support network will vary in size and composition; may be small and self-contained or may comprise many parts. Turnbull & Turnbull (1991) have proposed that the move to put disabled individuals and their families at the centre of the rehabilitation process (much as proposed by the approach in this book) rather than have them conform to the medical model of care and rehabilitation is not unlike the revolution in thinking caused by Copernicus when he put the Sun, rather than the Earth, at the centre of the Universe. Their work in applying a systems perspective to identify the individual strengths and needs of each family unit is based on earlier work in the field of learning disabilities.

Essentially Turnbull & Turnbull (1991) describe a framework to gain understanding based on four major components:

- Family characteristics
- Family interaction
- Family functions
- Family life cycle.

Characteristics is the description of the family, their strengths and limitations as a whole and as individuals. *Interaction* refers to the normal daily and weekly relationships within the family unit, how much contact they have, what type of contact, and so on. *Functions* relate to responsibilities and roles that individual members assume to meet their own needs and the wider needs of the family unit. Finally, *life cycle* looks at expected developmental changes such as children leaving the family home and other variables, for example in financial income or outgoings.

While most physiotherapists will not find themselves in the position of formally assessing family systems, this structure is useful to guide thinking in terms of potential barriers to implementing a preferred intervention or in identifying a family strength that could assist the implementation of a novel or more innovative approach to achieve the desired therapeutic outcome.

Awareness of these issues will also help therapists to appreciate more readily the sometimes complex set of circumstances being dealt with by social work colleagues or others who find themselves in an advocate role, for example an independent case manager.

The wider community

At the inpatient stage, the injured individual is usually quite removed from the influences of wider cultural and community factors, and the structure and process of the hospital culture sets the context for their behaviour. In normal circumstances visitors also adhere to the rules of the hospital environment and take guidance from hospital staff. When the person with a TBI returns home, the message is that they are no longer ill and the regulatory, sometimes prohibitive, hospital rules are replaced with normal freedoms and a level of expectation in terms of returning to regular social activities.

Gauging the optimum speed and level of attempting to return to previous activities is a difficult and inexact process. It is also a process that may be complicated by cultural misunderstandings on the part of professionals or by the ignorance of social contacts.

There may be unrecognized pressures to return to life management or social roles, for example to care for children or to re-establish the weekly night out at the pub. These pressures may run parallel to the individual's personal goals and, if poor judgement leads to an overestimation of capabilities, the potential for failure is high.

It is rarely realistic or feasible to provide direct education for the majority of even routine social contacts and yet successful community reintegration is often dependent upon the attitudes and understanding of just these people. One possible solution is to provide social contacts with appropriate information via the injured person or the immediate family, but this is often unacceptable for a variety of reasons. An alternative is to encourage the injured person to anticipate difficult situations involving more peripheral contacts and to prepare for them within the rehabilitation programme.

No matter what combination of these or other approaches is taken, the pivotal nature of those immediately affected by the trauma is again highlighted. It also follows that it is necessary to assist them, wherever possible, to understand the reality of their situation so that they can adjust in order to make honest and realistic decisions about tasks and activities that are appropriate to attempt. Where the injured individual has particularly poor judgement, the primary carer can find themselves in a buffer position in an effort to protect their loved one, and this function brings with it the potential for substantial friction in other aspects of their relationship.

In addition to formal health and social care provision there are, in all developed countries, specific self-help groups and campaigning organizations that can help with the educative, supportive and listening process. These organizations, for example Headway in the UK and in parts of Australia, and the National Head Injury Foundation in the USA, have produced useful publications and offer a variety of locally based services.

Many people find great support in being part of these groups, but for some being associated with others with disabilities is too painful to contemplate.

Within the wider community there is also much potential for support and assistance in achieving acceptable intervention outcomes. My own experience is that educative establishments, sports and exercise facilities, voluntary organizations and many other organizations external to the health or disability networks have the will and the ability to accommodate the special needs of those recovering from TBI if given adequate explanation, appropriate direction and support. If a good match is made between the capabilities of the individual and the demands of the activities to be undertaken, the successful outcome of their first experience facilitates their openness to assisting in a similar way in the future.

CONCLUSION

TBI has an impact on the lives of many people beyond the injured individual. In the early stages, especially in severe injury, the needs of carers in terms of support and information are paramount. The long-term nature of the recovery, rehabilitation and adjustment process demands that therapists working in the acute sector think beyond the immediate presenting problems and anticipate how they may contribute to the process as a whole.

Each individual affected will learn about, understand and adjust to the new situation at varying rates. Therapists need to understand the experience and process through which clients and carers are moving, be able to recognize the current stage and adjust their own expectations to take account of these factors. In recognition of the complex set of adjustments required of all that are affected, service provision should plan to deal with the predictable issues in a practical way. This is likely to mean therapists undertaking some of the routine counselling work in parallel with other discipline specific goals. In order to do this therapists must gain appropriate training and have ongoing advice and supervision from specialist psychological and social work colleagues.

Therapists must consider the appropriateness of the considered intervention at any particular time. This may include whether or not physiotherapeutic intervention is warranted, whether it is the priority for the client at that time, whether having discussed all the issues with other team members it is the priority for the team at that time, whether all the necessary support services are in place to allow therapeutic gains to be applied or maintained, and many other influencing factors.

Therapists should not lose sight of the need for carers to have a life of their own and, while it may be expected that they will want to contribute to care and rehabilitation programmes, their contribution should never be presumed. Accommodation to change in the longer term may well be facilitated by everyone involved having a degree of independence from one another, and certain therapeutic goals will be achieved only if the functional goal is seen by all as being the responsibility of the individual. Getting all of this right requires close liaison with the whole family unit to achieve consistency of aims and approach.

Injured individuals are rarely able to identify realistic long-term goals until the process of adjustment is well advanced, and they will require help in setting meaningful short-term goals during the process of recovery and rehabilitation. Acceptable goals are easier to identify if therapists have a working knowledge of the client's preinjury lifestyle and personal characteristics.

A major key to establishing cooperative working, assisting adjustment and fitting people to cope in the longer term is the early and ongoing provision of factual information and honest projections. With appropriate knowledge, carers and individuals can be active participants in the rehabilitation process, making a positive contribution, knowing that they are doing so, and developing confidence in coping.

Appropriate knowledge will also allow people to know the limits of their ability to cope so that they can anticipate their own needs or the needs of those dependent on them and ask for assistance from their own support network, voluntary or statutory services in good measure. When they are able to do this, they will have taken back control of their lives.

REFERENCES

Beaver M 1991 Special issues for a spouse. In: Williams J M, Kay T (eds) Head injury: a family matter, 1st edn. Paul H Brookes, Baltimore, MD, p 19

Brooks D, McKinlay W 1983 Personality and behavioural changes after severe blunt head injury – a relatives' view. Journal of Neurology, Neurosurgery and Psychiatry 46:336–344

Brooks D, Campsie L, Symington C, Beattie A, McKinlay W 1987 The effects of severe head injury on patient and relative within seven years of injury. Journal of Head Trauma Rehabilitation 2(3):1–13

Cavallo M M, Kay T, Ezrachi O 1992 Problems and changes after traumatic brain injury: differing perceptions within and between families. Brain Injury 6(4):327–335

Douglas J 1996 Indicators of long-term family functioning following severe traumatic brain injury in adults. Brain Injury 10(11):819–839

Douglas J M 1990 Traumatic brain injury and the family. Making headway: proc. NZSTA Conference, Christchurch, New Zealand

Fleming J M, Hassell M, Strong J 1996 The nature of impairment of self-awareness of deficits in severe traumatic brain injury. In: Ponsford J, Snow P, Anderson V (eds) International perspectives in traumatic brain injury. Australian Academic Press, Melbourne, p 438

Frosch S, Gruber A, Jones C et al 1997 The long term effects of traumatic brain injury on the role of caregivers. Brain Injury 11(12):891–906

Gleckman A D, Brill S 1995 The impact of brain injury on family functioning: implications for subacute rehabilitation programmes. Brain Injury 9(4):385–393

Goldberg D, Williams P 1988 A user's guide to the general health questionnaire. NFER-Nelson, Windsor

Hardgrove H 1991 Special issues for a child. In: Williams J M, Kay T (eds) Head injury: a family matter, 1st edn. Paul H Brookes, Baltimore, MD, p 25

Hopewell C A, Jackson H F, Jones W B 1989 Family support groups for traumatically brain injured patients. Dallas Neuropsychological Institute, Dallas, TX

Horowitz M, Wilner N, Alvarez W 1979 Impact of Event Scale: a measure of subjective stress. Psychosomatic Medicine 41:209–218

Junque C, Bruna O, Mataro M 1997 Information needs of the traumatic brain injury patient's family members regarding the consequences of the injury and associated perception of physical, cognitive, and emotional and quality of life changes. Brain Injury 11(4):251–258

Kramer J 1991 Special issues for a parent. In: Williams J M, Kay T (eds) Head injury: a family matter, 1st edn. Paul H Brookes, Baltimore, MD, p 9

Leaf L E 1993 Traumatic brain injury: affecting family recovery. Brain Injury 7(6):543–546

Leatham J, Heath E, Wooley C 1996 Relatives' perceptions of role change, social support and stress after traumatic brain injury. Brain Injury 10(1):27–38

Livingston M G, Brooks D, Bond M 1985 Patient outcome in the year following severe head injury and relatives' psychiatric and social functioning. Journal of Neurology, Neurosurgery and Psychiatry 48:876–881

McKinlay W W, Brooks D N, Bond M R, Martinage D P, Marshall M M 1981 The short-term outcome of severe blunt head injury as reported by relatives of the injured persons. Journal of Neurology, Neurosurgery and Psychiatry 44:527–533

McLaughlin A M, Carey J L 1993 The adversarial alliance: developing therapeutic relationships between families and the team in brain injury rehabilitation. Brain Injury 7(1):45–51

Marsh N V, Kersel D A, Havill J H, Sleigh J W 1996 Components of caregiver burden at six months following severe traumatic brain injury. In: Ponsford J, Snow P, Anderson V (eds) International perspectives in traumatic brain injury. Australian Academic Press, Melbourne, p 475

Novack T A, Richards J S 1991 Coping with denial among family members. Archives of Physical Medicine and Rehabilitation 72:521

Novack T A, Bergquist T F, Bennett G, Gouvier W D 1991 Primary caregiver distress following severe head injury. Journal of Head Trauma Rehabilitation 6(4):69–77

Oddy M 1995 He's no longer the same person: how families adjust to personality change after head injury. In: Chamberlain M A, Neumann V, Tennant V (eds) Traumatic brain injury rehabilitation: services treatments and outcomes. Chapman & Hall, London, p 167

Oddy M, Humphrey M, Uttley D 1978 Stresses upon the relatives of head-injured patients. British Journal of Psychiatry 133:507–513

Perlesz A, Kinsella G, Crowe S 1996 Family psychosocial outcome following traumatic brain injury. In: Ponsford J, Snow P, Anderson V (eds) International perspective in traumatic brain injury. Australian Academic Press, Melbourne, p 470

Ponsford J 1995 Working with families. In: Ponsford J, Sloan S, Snow P (eds) Traumatic brain injury: rehabilitation for everyday adaptive living, 1st edn. Lawrence Erlbaum, Hove, p 265

Prigatano G P, Altman I M 1990 Impaired awareness of behavioural limitations after traumatic brain injury. Archives of Physical Medicine and Rehabilitation 71:1058–1064

Prigatano G P, Fordyce D J 1986 Cognitive dysfunction and psychosocial adjustment after brain injury. In: Prigatano G P, Fordyce D J, Zeiner H K, Roueche J R, Pepping M, Wood B C (eds) Neuropsychological rehabilitation after brain injury. Johns Hopkins University Press, Baltimore, MD, p 1

Rees R 1988 How some families cope and why some families do not. Journal of Head Trauma Rehabilitation 3(3):72–77

Rimel R W, John A J, Bond M R 1990 Characteristics of the head injured patient. In: Rosenthal M, Griffith E, Bond M, Miller J (eds) Rehabilitation of the adult and child with traumatic brain injury, 2nd edn. FA Davis, Philadelphia, PA, p 8

Romano M D 1974 Family response to traumatic head injury. Scandinavian Journal of Rehabilitation Medicine 6:1–4

Rose F, Johnson D 1996 Brain injury and after: towards improved outcome, 1st edn. John Wiley, Chichester, UK

Rosenbaum M, Najenson T 1976 Changes in life patterns and symptoms of low mood as reported by wives of severely brain injured soldiers. Journal of Consulting Clinical Psychology 44:881–888

Rosenthal M 1989 Understanding and optimising family adaptation to traumatic brain injury. In: Bach-y-Rita P (ed) Traumatic brain injury, 1st edn. Demos Publications, New York, p 191

Talbott R 1989 The brain-injured person and the family. In: Wood R, Eames P (eds) Models of brain injury rehabilitation, 1st edn. Chapman and Hall, London, p 3

Telford R, Wright J 1992 Sheffield head injury survey. Sheffield Health Authority, Sheffield

Telford R, Wright J C 1996 Long-term consequences of minor head injury on family members. Clinical Rehabilitation 10:255–258

Turnbull A P, Turnbull H R 1991 Understanding families from a systems perspective. In: Williams J M, Kay T (eds) Head injury: a family matter, 1st edn. Paul H Brooks, Baltimore, MD, p 37

Tyerman A 1991 Counselling in head injury. In: Davis H, Falklowfield L (eds) Counselling and communication in health care. John Wiley, Chichester, UK, p 115

Williams J M 1991 Family reaction to head injury. In: Williams J M, Kay T (eds) Head injury: a family matter, 1st edn. Paul H Brookes, Baltimore, MD, p 81

The assessment process

SECTION CONTENTS

4

Initial considerations in the process of assessment

Key Points

- Assessment should be tailored to meet the objectives of each individual service but should also include the recording of information required by subsequent service providers
- Key influencing factors in defining the scope of assessment include injury severity, time postinjury, projected length of contact, remit of the service and the representation of other disciplines
- The gathering and synthesis of information concerning preinjury status and postinjury progress are crucial to defining the appropriate detail of an individual assessment
- Assessment should allow discrimination between desirable and achievable goals, and may lead to the conclusion that intervention is not appropriate
- There are a variety of assessment methods available and each method generates different types of data; TBI assessment should draw on all methods as appropriate to the type of information that is sought
- TBI assessment should be recognized as dynamic and ongoing but the assessment process can be streamlined and facilitated by methodical discussion and pre-planning across all potential contributors

INTRODUCTION

The previous two chapters of this book were designed to provide the reader with two main pillars of background knowledge from which to develop their approach to those referred for therapy services following TBI.

First, the potential scope of the injury and its subsequent effects were presented in parallel with management and documentation issues judged to have value in theoretical and practical terms. The details of the pathological process, medical interventions, and strengths and limitations of methods of assessment were given to enable therapists to be independent in their understanding and analysis of each individual's progress. With this knowledge therapists should have a baseline for evaluation of each individual's progress in the acute stage, allowing informed clinical discussion and decision making with regard to intervention design and information giving. It should also allow therapists responding to referrals in the post-acute stage to glean an accurate picture of an individual's initial status and progression from retrospective review of acute medical and therapeutic notes and, in so doing, contribute to informed goal setting and anticipation of potential outcome.

Second, the previous chapter encouraged therapists to take time out from the professional action role to consider the position and viewpoint of the injured person and that of their family and friends. This process was defended as being relevant in achieving service delivery that is perceived as good by those receiving it, and also essential in limiting inefficient use of resources in the form of pursuing inappropriate goals.

Knowledge of the severity of initial injury and subsequent progress, and understanding of individual characteristics, are essential components in outlining the scope of enquiry that is referred to as the assessment process. Having introduced the need to be knowledgeable with regard to these issues, this chapter will highlight some of the specific aspects that hold importance for developing an assessment process template. After consideration of some of the other influencing factors, for example place and time of contact, an outline structure for the assessment process will be proposed. We will then consider some of the practical issues to be considered by a service wishing to adopt this type of approach to assessment.

WHY IS ASSESSMENT A PROCESS?

The term *assessment process* is used to underline that assessment following TBI is not a one-off event. Even if we consider the physiotherapist's assessment at a single discipline level, in contrast to that which occurs as part of some kind of multiprofessional provision, the assessment should comprise much more than the face-to-face physical evaluation.

We will return to the question of defining the scope of information to be gathered later in this chapter, and in the following chapter go on to describe this in detail and explore potential information sources. But first we need to consider the factors that will strongly influence what kind of assessment is indicated.

The most obvious influence will be the type of service provision within which the therapist is working, and the following discussion is therefore structured to allow differences to be considered at the level of service provision, rather than at the level of assessment of the individual. Clinical examples will be employed to illustrate some of the salient points.

THE ASSESSMENT PROCESS IN ACUTE CARE

As with all acute provision, speed of response and accuracy of intervention require a concise and focused assessment. Physiotherapists working in acute traumatic brain injury (TBI) have two major treatment foci: respiratory health and physical management. Each intervention requires review and assessment of medical and nursing observations before treatment, along with personal assessment of status via, for example, bronchial auscultation or analysis of resistance to passive stretch.

The objectives of direct intervention – the promotion of respiratory health and the management of the physical manifestations of the TBI – remain constant wherever the injured individual is encountered. However, the ease with which medical and nursing observations can be accessed and the scope of primary information gathering required of the physiotherapist will vary depending on the type of ward or unit.

There are two main factors that differentiate the scope of the physiotherapeutic assessment in acute care. The first is whether or not therapists are working within a specialist facility and the second, and sometimes related factor, is how their role is defined within the healthcare team.

The specialist facility

Physiotherapists are likely to encounter patients with TBI in one of two main specialist facilities. The first is the neurosurgical unit and the second is either a general or other specialty intensive care unit (ICU). Within the former there will commonly be care protocols that will aid the speed and automatic nature of early assessment and intervention. These are likely to include guidelines for positioning, turning, interventions likely to influence intracranial pressure, and so on. So, in the direct provision of early care, the process of assessment and evaluation of intervention is likely to have a preordained structure.

There are many advantages of working within guidelines that are based on knowledge of the pathological process and that have been developed via previous research and evaluation. However, one of the dangers is that issues of individuality, as described in Chapter 3, may be less tangible and unthinkingly ignored in preference to routine response. This is more likely to occur where demand on the service is high, and in these circumstances accurate knowledge of past medical, social and family history becomes an important aspect of the wider physiotherapy assessment.

Baseline outcome following brain trauma is dependent on the preinjury condition of the brain, the primary damage caused by the impact and the secondary damage resulting from the ensuing pathological process (Miller 1982), and these same three criteria can equally be applied to the musculo-skeletal system. Thus, knowledge of a patient's preinjury history of drug misuse, or previous TBI, for example, should temper predictions to the family of positive outcome, while awareness of a previous compound tibial fracture may be an indicator to give particular consideration to proactive preventive casting of the lower limb.

Physiotherapists' assessment role on a non-neurosurgical ICU is likely to vary from that within the neurosurgical unit because of their different role within the care team. While it is likely that specialist medical management advice will be available from neurosurgical colleagues, the physiotherapist is likely to have to take a lead role in the day-to-day management of the physical consequences of the neurological insult. Thus, physiotherapists on a general ICU may find themselves, contrary to what might be expected, taking a more overt role as adviser to the rest of the healthcare team than might be the case where other team members have experience and knowledge of neurological dysfunction.

It is important to note a further potential assessment role for all therapists working in acute provision, which is that of assessment with reference to potential long-term physical effects and functional outcome. This role is probably more easily recognized within subacute provision but, as other acute team members are primarily focused on the present via their life-preserving and immediate care roles, therapists are well placed to evaluate intervention needs from a more longitudinal perspective. This role may be simply to counter the viewpoint that appropriate repositioning or reapplication of splints are relatively unimportant parts of the nursing care regime, or it may be to positively encourage aggressive treatment of long bone fractures in cases when the prognosis appears poor.

The effects of failing to do the latter are exemplified by the case of Darren (Case example 4.1).

Case example 4.1   Darren

At the age of 17 years, Darren sustained an extremely severe TBI in a motorbike accident. During neurosurgery a substantial part of one cerebral hemisphere had to be removed and he was ventilated for more than a month. Darren was not expected to live, and his closed femoral fracture was not reduced or realigned.

Darren was transferred to his local hospital where he was given a bed on an orthopaedic ward, but as his Glasgow Coma Score remained below 8 for a further 4 months he was not treated actively. Family endeavours resulted in him being transferred to a rehabilitation facility where, after many months of inpatient and outpatient therapy, he made sufficient progress to take a place at a specialist residential college for young people with TBI.

However, Darren did not progress even to independent standing as his femoral torsion was such that over the period spent in the orthopaedic ward he developed adductor–flexor spasticity with associated soft tissue changes including a substantial knee flexion deformity, which later could not be overcome.

The non-specialist facility

Beyond the ICU, or for those whose injuries do not require medical and nursing intervention at the level of the ICU, many people with a closed TBI, at least in the UK, will initially be cared for on a ward with staff whose specialist knowledge is in a field other than neurorehabilitation. As has been outlined in relation to ICU provision, this may well bring additional assessment responsibilities to physiotherapists delivering the routine provision on these wards.

In such cases it may be useful to approach the assessment process not from the normal standpoint of designing the therapeutic intervention but from the point of view of establishing whether or not the assessing therapist has the knowledge and skills required to deliver the necessary provision. This decision may depend on the availability of advice or support from other therapists. However, it may be that the physiotherapist does have the expertise to deliver provision appropriate to their own discipline's specialisms but that other important aspects of the desired care package, such as support for families, may be lacking.

Physiotherapists commonly respond to difficult circumstances by attempting to give the best possible care. It is important that they also learn to include in their assessment the question of whether the injured individual's global needs are best met by pursuing direct intervention in the face of other resource limitations or by facilitating onward referral to a more appropriate treatment facility. Where onward referral is not an option, the standard of care may be improved by accessing specialist assessment and advice in relation to the care of the individual and in order to provide appropriate levels of information and support for the family.

Summary of possible assessment components in acute care

This list summarizes the main component parts and potential scope of the assessment process in which the physiotherapist working in acute care may legitimately become involved:

- Assessment framed by protocols or guidelines
- Assessment for respiratory intervention
- Assessment for physical management and prevention of secondary damage
- Assessment to develop prognostic indicators
- Assessment to identify unmet needs
- Assessment for discussion with, or referral to, other professionals (health, social work, education) for immediate action
- Assessment for referral to other professionals for later action.

THE ASSESSMENT PROCESS IN SUBACUTE PROVISION

It is to be hoped that physiotherapy assessment in subacute provision takes place in the context of a wider team assessment. The necessary scope of responsibility for aspects of the wider assessment will probably depend on the composition of the team and to what extent there is common access to the assessment findings of each team member. As far as the scope of the sensorimotor assessment is concerned, it is worthwhile considering the potential use of information gathered at this stage.

Most immediate will be the need for assessment to define the treatment approach and content. However, the assessment of physical status also has potential usefulness beyond the immediate application of its findings to inform direct intervention. This baseline of sensorimotor strengths and deficits may prove useful to therapists involved at a later stage – even years later. If assessment is repeated at intervals, it could help to describe a changed profile over time. Such information would be invaluable in monitoring resolution of deficits or development of compensatory habits and, furthermore, analysis of the documented changes would shed some light on the thorny question of rate and continuity of physical recovery following TBI.

Another factor for consideration in designing the sensorimotor assessment in the subacute stage is the anticipated length of contact time and the likely, or desired, progress to be achieved within that timeframe. The most obvious example would be recognition of the need to limit the scope of assessment when contact is likely to be only a few days, while taking the responsibility to document status and progression fully if the inpatient stay is anticipated to extend to weeks.

Finally, while it may be clear to the treating therapists and other team members that physical progress has been achieved, and what the level of that achievement is, the assessment of status at the point of discharge is sometimes absent and, when present, is often lacking in precision. Statements such as 'partially resolved right-sided weakness' or 'improved balance' can be interpreted in a variety of ways depending on the bias of the reader and the starting point of the patient.

Therapists working in inpatient care are likely to be aware of the importance of their role in moulding the potential functional recovery for their patients, and in practice this is a responsibility that they take seriously and tackle well. However, it is not necessarily the case that they will understand the importance of their observations to other professionals who may be involved at a later date. Records of assessment and evaluation of progress may hold valuable information that can be observed only at that particular time. Precision in recording, including an indication of the context and focus of assessment, will aid the understanding of others and, sometimes more importantly, avoid misinterpretation.

The latter point can be a particular issue in the medicolegal context and since, in the UK, this is likely to affect around 75% of those sustaining TBI (Centre for Health Service Studies 1998), it is a matter for serious concern. For example, while therapists might interpret a recording of 'fully mobile' in the context that they suspect it was written (i.e. in the context of moving around a hospital ward), insurers can, and do, assume that this means without limits to mobility in the community. The practice of stating the context in which the assessment took place, or indicating exactly what was and was not tested, may reduce the potential for misunderstanding.

THE ASSESSMENT PROCESS IN POST-ACUTE PROVISION

Post-acute physiotherapy provision may be provided as part of a specialist team or at a single discipline level, and service referrals may be received from a variety of sources and at any time after the original injury.

The type of service will firstly influence the objectives of the assessment. For example, the service offered by a specialist outpatient team who operate as planned follow-up provision from an inpatient programme will be quite different from that provided by physiotherapists working within a specialist educational establishment. The objectives in the former case may relate closely to goals set during the inpatient stay, whereas objectives in the latter case would clearly need to be set in the context of the reasons for attending the educational establishment.

During inpatient provision, the severity of injury and progress to date is either known by therapists or easily accessible via review of the clinical notes. In the community, referrals may at best come with a brief medical and therapeutic summary and, at worst, with little more than a diagnosis. Because of the nature of their injuries, people who have sustained a TBI will have limited recall of their hospital stay and for this and many other reasons will be poor historians. Despite this, many therapeutic assessments rely on taking a history from the injured person.

When therapists receive an inpatient referral they do not visit the patient's bedside without first examining the medical and nursing records relating to the admission; those notes routinely include a summary of past medical history and present social history. When therapists work without the supporting structure of the hospital environment, they should have at least the same level of knowledge about the person who has been referred. Thus, before direct contact is made, therapists should access and record the relevant facts from the inpatient stay and, if time has elapsed since discharge, attempt to trace notes relating to any intervening therapeutic input or medical follow-up.

There is much information to be gleaned from this process and, although it may be time consuming and cause a little delay in making the initial contact after receiving the referral, it is an efficient use of the time invested. There are subcomponents of information that are of particular use at specific times after injury or in specific circumstances; some of these are highlighted below.

Early post-acute provision

When assessing someone who has recently been discharged from inpatient care, as well as being able to ascertain the severity of the injury and mapping the course of recovery, it is also useful to know, for example, how many transfers within and between hospitals occurred during the inpatient stay. It is useful to know whether all the inpatient period was spent close to the family home or whether substantial family travel has been involved. Knowledge of the particular hospital units where care was received gives therapists a picture of the style and content of that care.

Other specific information should also be recorded in the notes, for example whether families were given grave predictions about outcome. All of this knowledge allows therapists to prepare to meet the injured person and their family at the right level and with appropriate expectations.

The time that has elapsed since injury and the time since hospital discharge will also give a rough indication of where people might be in terms of the process of adjustment. For example, if there has been little time at home, there will not have been sufficient opportunity to try to return to all preinjury activities and, therefore, even carer reports of functional level may be incomplete or inaccurate.

Some previous knowledge of the individual's primary activity at the time of injury can also aid assessment planning. For example, the assessment of a university student should anticipate the enquiry of whether they are likely to be able to return to their course in the near future. A sales representative whose work extends over a wider geographical area will want to know about the possibilities for returning to driving.

Both of these clinical examples pose a question, the response to which is dependent on much more than physical factors, and this would arguably be the case in considering any question of functional outcome.

In more than a decade of post-acute practice I have not encountered one individual who had physical deficits without concomitant cognitive or behavioural problems. It seems self-evident that physical rehabilitation at this stage of the recovery process should always be set in the context of wider provision, at least at the level of assessment and the application of that assessment in terms of goal setting and treatment design. Ideally, the delivery of a physical programme should take place with the backup of, and in collaboration with, a full interdisciplinary team.

Other community provision

As the period between injury and referral increases, the preassessment gathering of information can become more crucial. In the early post-acute period it is relatively easy to trace the course of recovery and involvement with other services. Referrals are likely to come from hospital personnel and the implicit intent behind the referral for assessment still relates to exploring the potential for return to preinjury lifestyle.

When referrals are received a substantial time after hospital discharge, the objectives of the referral cannot be assumed to be the same as in the early post-acute period. The individual who has been referred may not have had previous access to community-based rehabilitation, or they may have had involvement with a whole variety of service providers.

If other services have been involved, it is important to find out both the scope and the outcome of their contact. Someone who has had repeated periods of contact with therapists with positive outcome may simply be in need of regular professional input. However, another person may have had as many service contacts, but with unsatisfactory outcomes. Closer examination of a case such as this might reveal a pattern of erratic attendance, which could have its root in inappropriate service design or be because of competing home and family demands. It is important to isolate the reasons and to control for these factors in advance of committing to a period of intervention.

In contrast, someone with multiple service contacts with a regular attendance record, but who still presents as dissatisfied with the outcome, may be experiencing difficulty in adjusting to a permanent impairment. Another person with a similar history may not have been able to apply successes achieved in therapy sessions to their real-life activity.

Case example 4.2   Ray

A colleague who was working as a senior physiotherapist in an outpatient neurophysiotherapy service contacted me for advice. She had recently received a referral from a general practitioner which asked for therapy intervention for a 40-year-old man named Ray who had a previous TBI and was described as having recently deteriorated in his walking ability.

What the referral did not mention was that Ray had sustained his injury as a teenager and had had no contact with services since hospital discharge 23 years earlier. Neither did it mention that Ray's father had died the previous year and his frail mother was finding it increasingly difficult to cope at home.

Within 4 weeks of him commencing a treatment programme, Ray's mother was admitted to hospital. Therapy sessions were soon taken up with discussions of how to pay the electricity bill, what to buy at the supermarket, and so on. Ray had also begun to phone the physiotherapist at other times in the week and it was his request for her to do some of his shopping that prompted the phone call to me.

Ray had never cared for himself or managed a home. He had not deteriorated in a truly physical sense; he had just stopped getting out and about because that was what he used to do with his father. He had no friends of his own and had transferred his dependence from his parents to his therapist. The general practitioner had made the referral without asking why Ray was less mobile and partly in an effort to give Ray's mother some respite.

The information gathered in each of these scenarios can be used to structure an appropriate response to the referral, which may include direct physiotherapeutic assessment, onward referral, or both.

Another dimension to consider in relation to late referrals is the source of referral and what factors contributed to the referral action, as is reasoned by Case example 4.2.

In the context of examining the full picture, the referral was clearly inappropriate, at least as the only course of treatment. My colleague unwittingly became Ray's social worker, occupational therapist, friend and counsellor, and, while physiotherapy would have made an appropriate contribution in a wider action plan to re-establish Ray's community mobility, no therapist could achieve the desired functional outcome with only physical intervention.

Late non-specialist provision

The need to ask some questions in advance of defining treatment goals and style of delivery applies equally to encounters between physiotherapists and individuals who have previously sustained a TBI, *no matter what the specialty area or treatment focus* is. People with a TBI are just as likely as other members of the general population to require, for example, the services of musculoskeletal specialists during their lives. And where neuromuscular deficits result in postural asymmetries or muscular imbalance, their need is likely to be greater.

Therefore, where part of a management programme, for instance for a lumbar spine problem, involves the patient in following management advice or contributing to their recovery by exercise, particular attention should be paid to the question of the individual's ability to follow and apply standard forms of education. If it is assumed that information processing, recall and self-directing skills are without fault, the expected progress will not be achieved. On the other hand, if the possibility of limitations in these areas is anticipated, the quantity and speed of information given, and the way in which it is given, can be adjusted and overt strategies for actioning practice can be developed.

Successful outcomes

All of the above descriptions were designed to illustrate the need to consider external influencing factors in an assessment process that begins at the point when a referral is received. It is a process that identifies and acknowledges a number of potential limiting factors in terms of successful therapeutic outcomes. It is part of a process that leads therapists to understand the difference between *desirable* and *achievable* goals and, importantly, what they might realistically expect to achieve as physiotherapists.

Conversely, the process can also help therapists understand why, despite their best efforts, some goals are not achieved, which is an extremely important issue in maintaining the motivation to continue working with this challenging group of clients and in changing practice to improve success in the future.

DEFINING THE SCOPE OF ASSESSMENT

What I have attempted to do so far in this book is to explain why it is important for physiotherapists to know and understand the wider issues associated with the pathology of TBI and the individual TBI victim. I have described medical, social and organizational factors that may directly or indirectly influence the outcome of physiotherapeutic intervention. Having presented the case for inclusion of these factors in the assessment process, I will now describe a structure and process that represents a clinically successful approach to assessment and intervention with this client group.

The assessment process, in particular, is drawn from my own and colleagues' extensive work to develop an efficient interdisciplinary assessment in the context of a specialist outpatient service. As a collaborative process, based in clinical practice, the contributors have been many, but I particularly acknowledge the personal contributions of my co-authors (Body et al 1996) in the paper that described the philosophy of the approach, which was published in the course of its development.

It is interesting to note that, although some minor changes have taken place in the years since this paper was written, the philosophy and component parts of the assessment report have remained relatively constant. It also feels important to stress that this has been the case even in the face of a number of staff and organizational changes. In fact the structure of the assessment process has, in my opinion, provided a level of consistency that would have been otherwise impossible to maintain during such a period of change.

I mention these issues to counter the idea that this approach to assessment, which on first reading may appear complex, is relevant only in the context of specialist interdisciplinary service provision. On the contrary, I would argue that the use of this structure, or a similar global template, allows all practitioners to think in holistic terms, even if it is only to the level of knowing that there are areas of potential influence about which they have no information. In such a case, the need for assistance from colleagues may be clearly identified, or the impossibility, as an independent practitioner, of meeting the objectives of the referrer or the goals of the individual can be stated in an objective manner.

DOCUMENTING A HOLISTIC ASSESSMENT

The following structure is therefore suggested as a working template from which to develop your own assessment protocol and within which to record your assessment findings. It is not suggested that a physiotherapist working as an independent clinician should necessarily be writing assessment reports covering all these areas. It is intended that, by being aware of the many aspects of potential deficit that will not be covered in a standard physiotherapeutic assessment, clinicians resist using language within their reports and in discussing assessment findings that implies normality in untested areas.

Applying the same thinking when considering the design and content of the physiotherapeutic intervention, therapists should avoid making inaccurate assumptions of individual's abilities, for example their ability to follow or remember complex instructions, to apply learning automatically in the home environment, or to negotiate time within the family to work on achieving goals. The details for inclusion under each heading and some methods of obtaining them are covered in the following two chapters and only a brief introduction is given here.

ASSESSMENT TEMPLATE
Background information

This should include:

- Medical information relevant to the traumatic event and the progress made to date

- Details of contact with other services
- Acknowledgement of the potential influence of relevant past medical history
- Current medication
- Medical and other review plans.

Lifestyle

This should give a picture of the person as an individual and include:

- An outline of previous and current personal history
- Practical aspects, such as living arrangements
- Details of work and leisure interests.

Psychosocial

This section should help describe present function and reported change with reference to:

- Mood
- Personality change
- Level of awareness of self and others
- Social interaction and relationships.

Core skills

As the title suggests, this section contains assessment findings that give information about the basic strengths and limitations an individual is working with, including:

- Attention and concentration
- Sensation and sensory processing
- Motor performance
- Language and communication
- Memory and learning.

Integration and organization

Having evaluated the basic building bricks, consideration is then given to the ability integrate and apply the core skills in a meaningful and self-directed way. This includes the ability to:

- Generate and develop realistic goals
- Plan and action activities to achieve identified goals

- Monitor performance during activities, recognizing and acknowledging errors
- Problem-solve to correct errors.

Life skills

Finally, this section describes what the individual *actually does* in terms of self-care, home management and wider community activities.

Summary and recommendations

Having taken into account all the assessment findings, the strengths and limitations identified can be summarized and the process of defining priorities for action and/or intervention begins. We will look at the process of defining goals for intervention in detail in Chapter 7.

PRACTICAL ISSUES

Having established the need to view physiotherapeutic intervention in the context of the natural pathology of TBI and its broad effects, and also with regard to the aspirations of the individual, it is necessary to describe the application of this approach in real and practical terms. We have already considered how to make use of preparatory thinking in order to decide on the realistic scope of assessment that should apply to each individual service.

The implication of following a process to define an optimum assessment is that assessments will, therefore, vary. It may then be viewed as somewhat contradictory to go on to describe a standard assessment process. However, the inclusiveness of the information presented is intended to describe a global matrix to support informed decision making with regard to what constitutes both the minimum acceptable and the optimum assessment standard for each service and for each individual case within that service.

The presentation of a holistic approach to assessment continues the theme of physiotherapists developing a wider knowledge base and, by making reference to specific cognitive assessments and other apparently peripheral information, also offers physiotherapists the opportunity to develop a better understanding of colleagues' work and of patients' experience.

While multiprofessional involvement in TBI rehabilitation is propounded as the 'gold standard' of care, there is surprisingly little space in the literature devoted to description of how to organize this type of working or to structure the recording of its product. Terms such as multidisciplinary, interdisciplinary and transdisciplinary are often used synonymously, whereas in fact they represent differing conceptual and organizational approaches.

In reality, although individual clinicians frequently come together to inform one another of their programme plans for individual clients via the format of the hospital ward meeting or clinical case conference, it is much less common to find the detailed discussion occurring in advance of the commencement of intervention. This is probably the primary difference between teams working on a multidisciplinary model and those embracing an interdisciplinary approach.

It is interesting to note that, as well as the assessment approach around which this description is structured, other guides to the process of effective assessment, treatment and recording that have emanated from specialist TBI programmes have all adopted an interdisciplinary (Children's Trust at Tadworth 1997, Powell et al 1994) or transdisciplinary (Jackson & Davies 1995) approach.

Using the basic assessment template headings to help structure the description of a complex process, Chapters 5 and 6 explore the scope of information to be gathered and describe ways in which it may be achieved. The emphasis in Chapter 5 is on the physiotherapist understanding and contributing to the global assessment, and in Chapter 6 the focus is on assessment areas of particular concern to the physiotherapist. The question of common and potential roles for the physiotherapist within an integrated approach to assessment is considered throughout both chapters.

The information-gathering process involves the use of a variety of assessment approaches and there is some discussion of the relative merits of each as they relate to the subsection under discussion. In advance of this, some of the vocabulary commonly used with reference to assessment will be introduced and explained, and then some of the practical considerations in moving towards an integrated assessment process will be addressed.

TYPES OF ASSESSMENT

Approaches to assessment are many and varied, and the information gathered may range from unsubstantiated report and subjective observation at one end of the spectrum to precise measurement at the other. How factual and relevant a piece of information is depends on the reliability and appropriateness of the information source, and on the quality of the information itself.

It is extremely important to understand these concepts of reliability, relevance and quality so that the information gathered is accurate and appropriate, and is interpreted and used in a meaningful way. Throughout Chapters 5 and 6, reference will be made to a number of different aspects of assessment which together comprise the full dynamic process; a brief description of each aspect is given below.

ASSESSMENT BASED ON SELF-REPORT

Sometimes termed 'subjective report', this aspect of assessment has value in that it comes directly from the individual being assessed and, in ideal circumstances, should alert therapists to areas of difficulty as seen from the viewpoint of the person who is having the problem. There is sometimes concern that reliance on self-report allows the individual with ulterior motives to claim problems that they do not have or to exaggerate symptoms they do have. In the course of normal assessment practice, however, the subjective report is used primarily to guide the scope and direction of assessment, and the physical or other objective examination of the therapist or doctor would be expected to elicit findings consistent with the self-report.

There are a number of specific reasons why it is inadvisable to place a heavy reliance on self-report in assessment following TBI. These reasons relate to the impact of cognitive dysfunction on the ability to (1) recognize, recall or report specific problems, and (2) anticipate the impact of deficits that are recognized on the ability to succeed in functional activities. Thus, the issue with those who have sustained a TBI is more usually a tendency to minimize rather than embellish reports of problems in response to open enquiry.

In a recent study this was found to be the case even in a group of 50 individuals pursuing compensation claims (Shordone et al 1998). However, self-report compared with carer report and contrasted with findings on objective assessment may be used, for example to define areas of poor awareness, which in itself can prove key in determining intervention plans and treatment goals.

ASSESSMENT BASED ON OBSERVATION

Much of the clinical assessment performed by neurophysiotherapists is observational or qualitative in nature. An individual's performance on a number of routine motor activities is assessed against the therapist's preconceived idea of normality. The validity of this approach is, of course, dependent on the model or models of *normality* that are used, and we will return to this later. Some structure may be afforded to the observational process by assessing and recording component parts of the function separately or by commenting on factors thought to underpin motor performance, for example sensory awareness, muscle tone and joint range of motion.

The problem with observational assessment that is not based on predefined criteria is that there is no way of knowing whether two therapists are measuring the same thing (interobserver reliability) or, indeed, whether the same therapist would rate in the same way on two different occasions (intraobserver reliability).

More formal structured observation can be achieved by using a checklist that both defines the behaviours to be observed and offers specific criteria to guide the rating. Put in simple terms, this at least means that everyone is looking at the same things and attempting to fit their observations into a narrow range of responses, for example present–absent or yes–no–sometimes.

More sophisticated rating scales may offer scope to record a wider range of responses. However, reliability studies looking at rating scales used in neurophysiotherapeutic practice have shown very poor inter-rater reliability when dealing with the nebulous concepts of muscle tone (Mayo et al 1991) and the validity of clinical tests of spasticity is also in question (Fowler et al 1998).

ASSESSMENT BASED ON STANDARDIZED INSTRUMENTS

Standardized assessments produce quantitative scores, which allow comparison with scores achieved by a standard, normal population, or enable the documentation of change over time, or both. Good standardized tests are developed to ensure consistent results independent of the person administering the test (reliability). They should also have been proven to test or measure what they claim to measure (content validity) so that deficits are not attributed where they do not exist and individuals are not pronounced deficit free when they do have problems. It is important to note, therefore, what populations have been used in validation studies and to remember, in interpreting the data gleaned from the assessment, what level or aspect of ability has been tested.

In tests that are formally published, information regarding reliability and validity, and the studies upon which these claims are made, will normally be recorded in the manual supplied with the test materials. It cannot simply be assumed that a formally published test is transferable to use with any pathology or age group, and it should be remembered that it is not the test itself that is 'validated', rather, the results of the test have been found to be valid for the population(s) tested.

In addition to these prepublication studies, and in common with those tests that are more freely available in the public domain, further investigations of reliability and validity should be published in peer-reviewed journals or presented at peer-assessed conferences or scientific meetings.

It is also crucial to understand the intended scope of a test. For example, an individual achieving a maximum score of 20 on the Barthel ADL (activities of daily living) Index (Mahoney and Barthel 1965) may be said to be independent of physical assistance in self-care activities but could not be presumed to be either free from physical restrictions or able to manage their own affairs completely. These latter assumptions may appear to be reasonable in the light of achieving a full score on an assessment with ADL in the title. However, examination of the content of the assessment reveals a bias towards the physical ability to achieve categories of self-care (using adaptations and adapted clothing if required) and does not test ability to perform any domestic activity of daily living such as washing or ironing clothes or preparing meals.

Therefore, the simple fact that a standardized test producing quantitative data is used within an assessment process does not mean that all questions regarding a particular deficit can be, or have been, answered. Moreover, it sometimes requires the administration of a number of assessments, focused on different aspects of the same issue, to inform the true functional meaning of data gathered from a single standardized test, and reasonable performance on a pen and paper test does not always mean that an individual can incorporate the skill tested into daily function.

Psychometric testing performed by psychologists and other therapists follows a process of clinical reasoning whereby a number of tests or subsections of tests are chosen on the basis of a variety of factors including the natural history of the underlying pathology and the individual's clinical presentation. The assessing clinician adapts and progresses the assessment dependent on the individual's performance and the end product, developed from a holistic analysis of resultant data, is a descriptive profile of their strengths and limitations, albeit based on tests that have on the whole been performed in a *controlled situation*.

Physiotherapists do not, on the whole, have the same history of assessing in this way. Neurophysiotherapists have barely got off the starting blocks in terms of the production of clinically acceptable tests of the underlying components of movement dysfunction. And, although some functional measures have found acceptance as gross measures of treatment outcome, their lack of specificity for treatment design means that they fail to produce the type of information that motivates busy clinical staff to adopt their use on a routine basis. More positive progress is being made towards the laboratory-research end of the evaluative spectrum, particularly with reference to kinematics and a variety of objective measures of muscle recruitment, activity and force generation.

We will come back to the question of the potential impact of using more standardized component-type assessments on treatment efficacy for physiotherapists. We will also look at the value of adopting, as a profession, a more cross-referencing approach to the analysis of movement dysfunction and the evaluation of treatment outcomes at the clinical interface, rather than pursuing the present apparently schizophrenic quest of, on the one hand, trying to perfect methods of assessing at impairment level, while at the same time recognizing the need to measure treatment outcomes as they relate to real-life function.

ASSESSMENT BASED ON RETROSPECTIVE REVIEW OF CLINICAL NOTES

The usefulness of gathering information about injury severity, previous medical and therapeutic intervention, speed of progression, and relevant past medical and social history was described in detail in Chapter 3. Indeed, the utility of gathering this type of information prospectively has long been an aspiration for experienced rehabilitation professionals for use in outcome evaluation and research, with a minimum data set for TBI now proposed in the USA (Hall 1997).

Chapter 2 outlined some of the necessary background knowledge of TBI pathology and methodological issues associated with assessments commonly used in acute care in order to allow appropriate retrospective interpretation of clinical recordings. In addition to these knowledge-related issues, consideration should also be given to the quality and reliability of other influential recordings.

Recordings made in an emergency facility are likely to be made under pressure of time. Shorthand phrases are frequently used, which by their nature do not allow for subtlety and so are open to misinterpretation. Thus a paramedic or triage nurse's observation of *smelling of alcohol* can easily become *drunk* and, without blood alcohol testing at the time, cannot later be quantified. In addition, recordings are usually based on the report of the individual (who may be concussed) or of the attending carer (who may be traumatized or anxious, or without full knowledge of the event or relevant medical history). Information may reach the medical assessor third-hand. For example, a witness to the incident passes information to the paramedic, who reports to the admitting nurse, who then appraises the doctor who makes the recording.

The clinical significance of understanding what actually occurred at the time of the incident is exemplified by the case of Tom (Case example 4.3).

ASSESSMENT BASED ON ALL OF THESE

From this brief overview it is apparent that none of these assessment methods constitutes the 'gold standard' on its own. Equally, a picture emerges that each method contributes a different type of information and has the potential to offer a particular perspective on a variety of issues. Therefore, any assessment that is carried out with the intention of gathering adequate information to develop a clear understanding of the individual presenting for advice or intervention should incorporate a number of assessment methods.

Case example 4.3   Tom

Tom's medical record stated that he had fallen over while drunk, thus sustaining a period of lost consciousness. From the original record, this statement was reiterated in the assessment of the admitting medical officer, in the transfer summary to inpatient rehabilitation, and in the referral to outpatient rehabilitation.

In fact, what had actually happened was that Tom, having been to the pub and consumed some alcohol, was standing outside chatting to two friends. Without warning he lost consciousness and fell, hitting the back of his head on the ground. Further discussion revealed that he had had a similar sudden loss of consciousness a few weeks earlier while sitting with some friends but had decided not to mention this to his wife so that she would not worry.

Tom was admitted by ambulance, called from the pub, without carer escort. When his wife joined him at the hospital, she reported no relevant past medical history and thus the assumption that he must have fallen over while drunk was not challenged.

Subsequently, the outpatient rehabilitation team also developed a suspicion of absence attacks based on further history gathered from the family, and when medical evaluation did not reveal another reason for his drop attacks he was commenced on anticonvulsant medication.

DYNAMIC ASSESSMENT

It may also be useful, at this point, to consider a further dimension of assessment, which we have not yet discussed. Assessment is acknowledged as being an important activity at the beginning of a new therapeutic relationship, but its role in the course of ongoing intervention is less clear. It is hoped that the subsequent text will be seen to be supportive of an approach to intervention that continues to gather information, evaluate response to treatment, and cross-reference findings across practitioners and disciplines. However, in trying to present information in a clear and unambiguous way, it may sometimes appear that assessment is being described only in relation to defining an initial baseline.

It is therefore stressed that all the principles and methods of information gathering that are described here and elsewhere in this book constitute a continuous and dynamic process, albeit with some more obvious milestones such as a baseline assessment or a discharge summary.

DEVELOPING THE MECHANICS OF ASSESSMENT

Before considering the detail of the assessment and how it might proceed, a primary decision needs to be made about the scope of assessment that is relevant to the design of the service and feasible within its resources. To design a new assessment process, or to rethink and revamp an old one, requires decisions to be made in four primary areas. Although they are presented here as occurring in a chronological way, in practice there is likely to be movement back and forward between each of the stages.

Ideally, such a development process should take place through discussion with a group of clinicians, with representation from a wide range of disciplines. In a new service, the foundation stage is to discuss and confirm the approach that will be adopted by the service as a whole. Beyond this there are interdependent questions of what level of detail of information is intended to be gathered, the design of the process within which this will happen, and by what means all of this will be achieved.

GUIDANCE OFFERED BY THE PHILOSOPHY OF THIS BOOK

We have already identified a number of factors as being important in determining an effective individual approach to our professional contact with those who have sustained a TBI; these can form the basis of the consideration of a collaborative service approach. They are:

- Try to place the client as an individual at the centre of your approach
- Acknowledge the wider impact of TBI and particularly its effects on family and friends
- Adopt a longitudinal approach, referring back for relevant information and forward to inform assessment and treatment planning
- Consider the remit of your service and your role within that service
- Reflect on what might be feasible within your resources
- Reflect on what might be possible if your resources were joined with others
- Be innovative in thinking about your role and remember that your objective is to provide the most relevant, efficient and effective intervention within the resources available to you.

QUESTIONS TO CONSIDER

If you as an individual, or your team as a whole, wish to revisit your approach to assessment, it may be helpful to consider some of the following practical questions.

What information do I need?

What is the core information set that will allow you to decide whether physiotherapeutic intervention would be appropriate, give you a basis upon which to suggest appropriate treatment goals and design the initial treatment strategies? How would you categorize the type of information you would want to gather? How much detail within each category do you need? How much is the information gathering process likely to be similar for each case and what, if anything, is likely to be different?

What information does my team need?

What is the relationship between the information that you, as an independent clinician, need and that which is required by other team members to inform their intervention plans? Are there things you all need to know? Is there information that you could gather that would be useful to other team members, and are others likely to be able to provide you with similar assistance?

What information is available to record now that will help in the future?

What are your (or your team's) responsibilities in terms of the full rehabilitation process? Can you help facilitate progress or understanding by ensuring clear recordings of key observations or information that will be useful for later service contacts? Or, in the case of post-acute services, can progress be facilitated by accessing and taking proper account of previously recorded information?

Can useful information be gathered from external sources?

Are there establishments or individuals who hold information that may inform your assessment? Are these sources likely to have been accessed before and, if so, will the information be collated in some way? Is there, then, a primary information source (such as a discharge summary) to access in the first instance?

How feasible is the gathering of information from these sources?

Can you gain access to the clinical notes or have copies of assessment, progress or discharge reports? How many institutions are involved and is it possible to get information from all appropriate sources?

OUTLINING THE ASSESSMENT PROCESS

When you begin to develop an idea of the scope of information you want to gather and you have addressed some of the issues raised by the preceding questions, it may then be useful to consider the potential for automation within the emerging process.

How much can be made routine or automatic?

Aspects of both the overall information gathering process and some of the direct assessment can be established as routine, without compromise to the principle of each assessment being focused and individual. For example, the process of trawling for previously recorded information can be structured in a logical order and targeted in a predetermined way. It may be that you decide, for instance, to access the records that you expect to be most informative first and to gather others only if there is missing information or need for clarification. If a consistent scope of information is to be gathered from carers, then a predesigned structured or semistructured questionnaire can be used, helping standardize the information gathered and easing the interview process. Many other forms of standardized documentation can be used in a similar way.

Can the process be made more efficient?

As well as adopting some routine practices within the overall process and using supportive documentation when gathering repetitive types of information, efficiency can be improved in other ways. For example, regular referrers can be supplied with referral forms that ask for a minimum data set such as demographic information, basic injury and medical details, addresses and contacts at involved institutions, names of involved professionals and discharge plans. Having agreed the remit of the service, criteria for acceptance to the service can be outlined and made available to referrers so that only appropriate referrals are received.

MAKING IT HAPPEN

None of the individual parts of this process has a distinct endpoint and it is useful to be aware that an *ideal assessment* is unlikely simply to emerge and be agreed. There is no predefined exact process, few universally agreed standardized assessments and many unanswered questions with regard to the majority of assessment dimensions that you will be considering.

At some point in the process, whether you are examining your practice as an independent clinician or as part of a wider team exercise, the decision has to be made to try to begin to put some of the agreed principles of the new or reworked assessment process into action. It may be useful to agree to do so for a time-limited trial period and to formalize the process of evaluation in some way in order to give status to the developmental process and ensure the experience is used constructively.

It may be only when attempts are made to action the process or to use a particular assessment that absolute decisions can be made as to whether the process is suitable to the purpose (or simply the best available at present) and whether or not it is feasible to use.

Who will collect what and how will we share the information?

Practical decisions relating to devolving responsibility for gathering sections of information and establishing mechanisms for sharing and cross-referencing the information *at an appropriate stage in the process* also need to be made in advance of testing out the system. If you are attempting to assess as a team, this involves the development of trust in colleagues to remember to collect all the information and to collect it in a way that will be as meaningful to you as if you had collected it yourself. It also involves establishing systems and processes to facilitate adequate communication and developing faith in those processes.

Where constituent parts of a service are not separated geographically, or when the physical barrier can be overcome by the application of information technology, the most logical focus for sharing information is to have a single case-note or patient record. The single patient record can range from being fully integrated, where recordings are entered consecutively one after the other, through those that have both communal and separate sections, to those that are simply a central storage-point for what are essentially single-discipline notes.

If your chosen assessment process involves collaborative information gathering or deliberate triangulation of the gathered data, the process needs to include a forum for exchange and discussion of the emergent data. As well as being a forum to structure the exchange of information about an individual client, this type of meeting should be regarded as an active part of the assessment process, where assessment findings are confirmed or reinterpreted in the light of additional information. In addition, as we still have limited understanding of how many of the frequently observed deficits fit together, this kind of focused discussion can help develop understanding and even generate hypotheses.

The success or otherwise of such a collaborative approach to assessment is dependent upon healthcare practitioners being willing and able to share their knowledge and to listen to others from an open, objective standpoint.

Relationships with other professionals

One of the many reasons I have chosen to strive for a client-centred approach to working is the clarity it gives when approaching the sometimes difficult questions and issues that arise from working in conjunction with many disciplines and many individuals within those disciplines. It is not always easy to achieve collaborative working and involvement in the process, as developing and sustaining this kind of approach may involve substantial personal challenges.

One of the frequently quoted barriers to true team working is said to be *professional jealousy* or *protectionist behaviour*, which is a complex issue that cannot be fully explored here. However, whatever factors motivate such behaviour need to be addressed in order that finite resources can be brought to bear on the complex and demanding issues encountered following TBI.

Clinical experience shows us that, even with all the specialist knowledge of the core professions involved in neurorehabilitation, there is so much that we do not yet know. With regard to the TBI population in particular, there are such huge needs that we as professionals barely begin to meet. We need to be constantly evolving our practice in the light of experience and evidence, and in the context of what constitutes the best service for the client group.

Physiotherapists have a unique body of knowledge to contribute to the team process and we have much to learn about the knowledge and practice of other discipline groups. There is tremendous potential for new learning when knowledge is shared, and the process of doing so should help us better to meet the needs of those we endeavour to assist.

Relationships with other services

It will help in defining your own assessment process to consider your relationship with other local services. If you are based in an acute hospital, this will be about other contributory services within the hospital and also institutions or community-based services to which onward referrals may be made. In addition to ensuring that your assessment includes the type of information sought by these other services, active consultation will have the effect of forging links that will facilitate more collaborative working in other areas of practice.

The families of those who have sustained a TBI frequently highlight the disjointed and disparate nature of the services they access as a primary concern. They find it difficult to understand why information they have given to the first or second service is not made available to the third and subsequent services.

If your service is post-acute, it may be worthwhile to consider the information needs of possible points of onward referral or discharge, for example relating to an employment placement, to facilitate function within an educational establishment or to assist ongoing function within the family or wider community.

Assistance from administrative and clerical staff

Finally in this section, the potential role of administrative, clerical and other support staff should be a definite consideration. Whether in relation to knowledge of information systems, the day-to-day smooth running of agreed processes, or as a first-level contact for those seeking information, there are many ways in which support staff can improve the quality, efficiency and effectiveness of a complex service.

REFERENCES

Body R, Herbert C, Campbell M, Parker M, Usher A 1996 An integrated approach to team assessment in head injury. Brain Injury 10(4):311–318

Centre for Health Service Studies 1998 National Traumatic Brain Injury Study. Warwick University, Warwick

Children's Trust at Tadworth, Rehabilitation Team 1997 Format and procedure for writing an interdisciplinary rehabilitation report. British Journal of Therapy and Rehabilitation 4(2):70–74

Fowler V, Canning C G, Carr J H, Shepherd R B 1998 Muscle length effect on the pendulum test. Archives of Physical Medicine and Rehabilitation 79(2):169–171

Hall K 1997 Establishing a national traumatic brain injury information system based upon a unified data set. Archives of Physical Medicine and Rehabilitation 78(suppl 4):S5–S11

Jackson H F, Davies M 1995 A transdisciplinary approach to brain injury rehabilitation. British Journal of Therapy and Rehabilitation 2(2):65–70

Mahoney R I, Barthel D W 1965 Functional evaluation: the Barthel index. Maryland Medical Journal 14:61–65

Mayo N E, Sullivan S J, Swaine B 1991 Observer variation in assessing neurophysical signs among patients with head injuries. American Journal of Physical Medicine and Rehabilitation 70(3):118–123

Miller J 1982 Physiology of trauma. Clinical Neurosurgery 29:103

Powell T, Partridge T, Nicholls T et al 1994 An interdisciplinary approach to the rehabilitation of people with brain injury. British Journal of Therapy and Rehabilitation 1(1):8–13

Shordone R J, Seyranian G D, Ruff R M 1998 Are the subjective complaints of traumatically brain injured patients reliable? Brain Injury 12(6):505–516

5

Understanding and contributing to the global assessment

Key Points

- Within an interdisciplinary model each discipline can have a wider role in gathering assessment information but effective information sharing and appropriate use of administrative assistance should mean a more efficient use of everyone's time
- There is a body of information required by all team members that should be gathered only once and shared across the team
- Some aspects of the global assessment lie outside physiotherapeutic core knowledge, but in developing an increased level of understanding of these areas physiotherapists will improve their overall standard of practice; an outline description of these wider aspects is given along with some examples of strategies for gathering information appropriate to each area
- There is potential for increased physiotherapeutic involvement in the gathering of information and the discussion of findings

ASSESSMENT DETAILS AND SOURCES OF INFORMATION

Using the structure of the assessment report introduced in Chapter 4 (see Fig. 5.1), we will now look at the sections of the assessment that would not

Background information
Lifestyle
Psychosocial
Core skills
Integration and organization
Life skills
Summary and recommendations

Figure 5.1 Template assessment report headings

normally be the primary concern of the physiotherapist and consider in some detail the type of information to be gathered. We will also consider the factors that influence methods of assessment and how responsibility for information gathering with respect to these headings may in some instances be divided across the team. Areas of assessment where the physiotherapist would expect to make a primary contribution are considered in more detail in Chapter 6.

BACKGROUND INFORMATION

CONTENT

Many of the data to be gathered, summarized and presented in this section are factual and static in nature and, at least in the gathering stage, can be assigned to someone with no clinical knowledge. The component parts will vary to accommodate the full history, depending on the stage following the injury at the point of service contact.

Thus, in acute provision, in addition to the mechanisms and results of the trauma, the history will be concerned with preinjury medical and social history. As more time elapses between the trauma itself and initial contact with particular services, information about the process and outcome of the preceding services also needs to be included.

MECHANISMS

Given the preceding comments with respect to detail and accuracy of subjective comment in clinical notes, it may be useful to incorporate some sort of confirmatory process, for example by asking a few standard questions of someone who (a) is knowledgeable about the injured person before the trauma, (b) was around in the immediate postinjury period, and (c) is knowledgeable about the path taken through the services.

In some cases the same person will fulfill each of these criteria but, for example in the case of a young person who has been living away from home, multiple informants may be required to obtain the whole picture. Clearly, if each service in turn recorded the salient points and passed them on, this process would be less time consuming, new services could be better prepared in advance of meeting families and individuals, and more time could be spent addressing the priority issues of the moment.

The primary mechanisms for gathering this type of information are semistructured interviews; review of notes, reports and discharge summaries; standard referral forms; and direct liaison with healthcare colleagues. In essence, the information presented should indicate clearly what has happened to bring the individual to this point and include the major medical influences from the past, such as any previous neurological or psychiatric history, and present influencing factors such as medication, planned medical review or potential surgical intervention.

In the post-acute period, the process of interviewing carers to expand or corroborate information found in the clinical notes (and usually to gather other information at the same time) offers an opportunity to gauge their level of satisfaction with progress to date and to develop an initial impression of their position along the process of adjustment (see Ch. 3).

Via this process it is also possible to describe the pattern of contact with services and, importantly, to highlight unsupported periods. Unlike the routine of gathering written or computer-generated information, the interview process demands a high level of clinical skill to glean the information required by the assessment process, to respond to the often difficult questions posed by the interviewee and, while doing so, to be able to offer sensitive and appropriate levels of support.

Within a team assessment, this type of interview can and should be carried out by clinicians from all clinical backgrounds. However, inexperienced clinicians will need education and coaching before doing so, and *all clinicians* may from time to time require debriefing following difficult or challenging sessions.

LIFESTYLE

CONTENT

There are two broad areas to be tackled in this section. The first is to try to give a clear representation of the individual before the trauma: to document sufficient information to develop a picture of their home, work and social life, their future plans and, where possible, to understand what constituted the important things in their life.

The second is to record any change in the basic organization or balance of these primary life roles that has occurred as a result of the injury and to indicate whether preinjury plans have been reconsidered or whether, at the point of assessment, they remain the same.

MECHANISMS

There are a variety of ways in which this type of information can be gathered, but in essence the majority of the data will need to come via the self-report of the individual and their carers. It is important, within a team context, to decide in advance who is responsible for gathering subsections of the information to ensure that all important areas are covered and no areas are unnecessarily duplicated.

It is also important to design the assessment process to take account of predictable consequences of the injury, such as post-traumatic amnesia, difficulties in organizing the presentation of information (e.g. presenting a work history in chronological order), possible confabulation, and so on. It is useful to ask the same questions of clients and carers (separately) and to include at least one observable test of a functional activity within the assessment so that conclusions about true activity levels can be made with greater confidence.

It is also useful to offer a structured checklist to record before and after frequencies of home- and community-based activities (Fig. 5.2). This is particularly useful in drawing attention to activities that have not yet been attempted (e.g. shopping, visiting the bank, using public transport) so that a distinction can be made between *no problems* and *no problems within limited activities*.

The choice of which practitioner gathers what information will be influenced by their need for information in order to progress other parts of their more specialized assessment. Thus, it makes sense for a psychologist to enquire about school grades and progress within formal education to assist in the choice of test materials. Likewise, occupational therapists will find a preamble related to activity levels in the home useful in preparing a functional task at an appropriate level. Physiotherapists will gain similar insights from gathering a leisure history.

The decision regarding the entire scope of information to be gathered by each team member will be influenced by these and other factors, such as the number of disciplines represented within your team, the overall quantity of information you are attempting to gather, the total time you can assign to the process, and the individual balance of time available depending on staffing levels and the quantity of assessment that is discipline specific.

PSYCHOSOCIAL

We have already discussed to some extent the reasons why it is important for all of us to understand how the injured individual is performing at a

PART 1

These questions are all about **before the injury**. Please tick the box under the heading that indicates (as nearly as possible) how often they would have been involved in EACH activity.

ACTIVITY	Every day	Several days per week	Once per week	Once per month	Once per year	Never
Tidying and light cleaning	☐	☐	☐	☐	☐	☐
Heavy household cleaning	☐	☐	☐	☐	☐	☐
Doing the laundry	☐	☐	☐	☐	☐	☐
Making snacks or hot drinks	☐	☐	☐	☐	☐	☐
Cooking main meals	☐	☐	☐	☐	☐	☐
Childcare or supervision of children	☐	☐	☐	☐	☐	☐
Planning meals	☐	☐	☐	☐	☐	☐
Managing finances	☐	☐	☐	☐	☐	☐
Reading for pleasure	☐	☐	☐	☐	☐	☐
Watching TV	☐	☐	☐	☐	☐	☐
Listening to music	☐	☐	☐	☐	☐	☐
DIY activities	☐	☐	☐	☐	☐	☐
Arts and crafts (e.g. needlework, woodwork)	☐	☐	☐	☐	☐	☐
Chatting	☐	☐	☐	☐	☐	☐
Playing with children	☐	☐	☐	☐	☐	☐
Using the local shops	☐	☐	☐	☐	☐	☐
Using larger stores	☐	☐	☐	☐	☐	☐
Shopping for clothes or personal items	☐	☐	☐	☐	☐	☐
Using the post office or bank	☐	☐	☐	☐	☐	☐
Travelling as a passenger in a car	☐	☐	☐	☐	☐	☐
Driving a car	☐	☐	☐	☐	☐	☐
Using public transport	☐	☐	☐	☐	☐	☐
Walking to local facilities	☐	☐	☐	☐	☐	☐
Sport or outdoor leisure	☐	☐	☐	☐	☐	☐
Visiting friends or relatives	☐	☐	☐	☐	☐	☐
Visiting the local pub	☐	☐	☐	☐	☐	☐
Having a night out	☐	☐	☐	☐	☐	☐

Figure 5.2 Part of an activity checklist to be completed by a carer

psychosocial level. We have, in particular, highlighted the futility of trying to press ahead without due regard to the individual's ability and readiness to engage.

As described by Tyerman (see Ch. 3), there are probably two main degrees of psychosocial impact on the normal rehabilitation process. The first is at the level at which general assistance to progress can be provided by the support of an experienced traumatic brain injury (TBI) clinician, irrespective of their discipline background. The second, where the impact is more complex, requires the specialist intervention skills of a clinical neuropsychologist.

Beyond this type of analysis, which is to some degree dependent on a fairly standard progression through reasonably responsive services, there are clients who, by the nature of their deficits or as a result of inappropriate or inadequate treatment, have developed disruptive or otherwise challenging behaviour. Individuals in the latter two categories will always require an initial period of highly specialized intervention, usually of a residential or 24-h nature.

It is probably quite useful to regard approaches to assessment in a similarly defined way and, in this respect, most of the following discussion applies primarily to people displaying the more common psychosocial dysfunctions and *only when therapists are supported within an interdisciplinary or transdisciplinary team including a clinical neuropsychologist.*

In stressing the potential for all team members to contribute to the assessment process, it is not the intention to minimize the role of the psychologist, even with regard to those individuals following a fairly recognizable path. While team members can certainly observe, report and discuss aspects of psychosocial behaviour as part of the initial and ongoing assessment process, the specific interpretation and definitive judgement regarding mood and behaviour is the province of the psychologist. In complex cases the psychologist may collaborate with psychiatric colleagues and particularly specialized assessment may be sought from a neuropsychiatrist.

This basic outline of potential grades of psychosocial dysfunction is given to assist therapists, particularly those without direct access to psychological services, in making the judgement of when they may initially proceed without specialized psychological assessment and, of equal importance, when it is correct to assert that their intervention is inappropriate without assessment and/or intervention from psychology colleagues.

The content and mechanisms given below under each subheading will also be of use in developing the reasoning that should underpin this decision process. The subheadings can also be used to aid team discussion and to help develop an appreciation of the impact of dysfunction in each of these areas.

MOOD

The first subheading is mood, which in this context covers all aspects of observed, reported and assessed affective (emotional) behaviour. Within this section there would be comment, for example, on any apparent variations from a standard behavioural presentation, specifically when these behaviours appear to be interfering with normal life activities or have the potential to block progression.

This type of information can be gathered by self and carer report (via semistructured interview), review of clinical notes and/or discussion with foregoing healthcare professionals, observation during the assessment period by all involved in the process, and direct assessment. Discussion of staff observations will be assisted by adding structure to the observations, either at the time of assessment in the form of a checklist of observed behaviours or at the time of discussion via a checklist of discussion points.

A variety of direct assessment scales looking at both general and specific aspects of mood have been developed, mainly in the mental health field. Some of these scales are complex and time consuming to administer or inappropriate for use with the TBI population for other reasons. However, there are a few short measures of general well-being, for example the General Health Questionnaire (GHQ 28) (Goldberg & Williams 1988), or those that screen for specific problems, for example the Hospital Anxiety and Depression Scale (Zigmond & Snaith 1983), which have found favour within general clinical practice.

PERSONALITY CHANGE

Personality change is a potentially difficult concept to deal with in terms of objective assessment since it is not often the case that the injured person would have been known to the assessing professional before the injury. It would also be extremely rare for there to be any record of personal attributes available to be used in a before and after measure. However, the high incidence of self- and carer-reported change in a variety of personal attributes across the whole spectrum of injury severity, and the significant impact of this type of change on individuals and family units, demands that careful consideration is given to this area.

One method of quantifying the perceived change is to ask the carer and the injured person separately to rate the injured person's personal attributes before and after the injury. This may be done using a set of semantic differentials as presented in Figure 5.3.

This procedure, which has been reported by Tyerman & Humphrey (1984), McWilliams (1991) and others, is easily incorporated into the semistructured interview already recommended. As well as informing the assessor, change recorded with respect to individual attributes can be used

Name of client: **Date:**

Please indicate on the five-point scale for each of the following 18 questions how you would describe yourself **after the injury** by placing a cross on each line.

1 Talkative	☐	☐	☐	☐	☐	Quiet
2 Even tempered	☐	☐	☐	☐	☐	Quick-tempered
3 Relies on others	☐	☐	☐	☐	☐	Independent
4 Affectionate	☐	☐	☐	☐	☐	Cold
5 Fond of company	☐	☐	☐	☐	☐	Dislikes company
6 Irritable	☐	☐	☐	☐	☐	Easy-going
7 Unhappy	☐	☐	☐	☐	☐	Happy
8 Excitable	☐	☐	☐	☐	☐	Calm
9 Energetic	☐	☐	☐	☐	☐	Lifeless
10 Down to earth	☐	☐	☐	☐	☐	Out of touch
11 Rash	☐	☐	☐	☐	☐	Cautious
12 Listless	☐	☐	☐	☐	☐	Enthusiastic
13 Mature	☐	☐	☐	☐	☐	Childish
14 Sensitive	☐	☐	☐	☐	☐	Insensitive
15 Cruel	☐	☐	☐	☐	☐	Kind
16 Generous	☐	☐	☐	☐	☐	Mean
17 Unreasonable	☐	☐	☐	☐	☐	Reasonable
18 Stable	☐	☐	☐	☐	☐	Changeable

Figure 5.3   Part of the process of defining changes in personal characteristics

to structure discussions with the informant(s), for example to validate their distress or for other illustrative reasons. Where ratings are obtained from both parties, comparison between perceptions can also be made.

AWARENESS

The third subheading covers awareness, both of matters relating to the client themselves and of the impact of circumstances and events on others.

Information and interpretation presented under this heading are developed from comparing self-report with the report of others and the findings on objective assessment, and are placed within the context of what might be reasonable to expect at the point of recovery. It is this context that will differentiate between:

- Lack of awareness borne out of limited experience of the impact of deficits
- Developing awareness in line with increasing experience of the impact of deficits
- Lack of awareness in spite of repeated experience of failure due to deficits
- Lack of awareness of the impact of their deficits and/or behaviour on others
- Full awareness of the impact of their deficits on themselves and others.

SOCIAL INTERACTION AND RELATIONSHIPS

Finally within this section, we consider social interaction and relationships. To some extent this is a summary of how all the previous sections are affecting daily behaviour and how that behaviour is cumulatively impacting upon significant relationships.

Whereas a variety of limited interactions may be observed during the assessment process, it is more difficult in the short term to obtain objective evidence of the status of relationships. Information may be available from social work colleagues or other professionals who have been involved in a counselling role. When there are distinct problems, friends or other family members may contact your service to volunteer information, express concern or seek guidance.

Observation of interactions between friends and carers contributing to the assessment process may also yield additional information. This may be a particularly rich source if part of the assessment is carried out in the family home when a larger number of people may be encountered.

ATTENTION AND CONCENTRATION

The ability to engage, sustain and disengage attention appropriate to the task in hand and to process the information generated within the task are all crucial for performance. Within this section of the assessment, structured observation and testing is directed towards identifying what aspects of attention, concentration and information processing are available and being used by the person being assessed and what aspects present barriers to specific functional tasks.

Where the individual is being assessed by a variety of practitioners in settings with varying levels of structure and differing levels of distraction, standardized observation can produce rich data. Problems may be observed in any or all of the following dimensions.

ENGAGING ATTENTION

Observations are sought with regard to the ability to engage attention to self-directed tasks, for example reading the newspaper while waiting to be seen, and to a variety of tasks within the assessment process. Differing performance levels may be noted depending on the apparent formality of the task, the amount of direction given, the perceived difficulty, or the level of interest or fatigue at any given time. Observations may also be made with regard to the appropriateness of completing or disengaging from a task and whether prompting or assistance is required to do so.

SELECTIVE ATTENTION

Another area of importance is whether or not the individual being assessed can hold their attention to the given or chosen task in the face of distraction. Some individuals may be distracted by their own thoughts or preoccupations. Specific cognitive deficits, such as difficulties in orientation or memory, may induce agitation, which acts as a barrier to attention. Similarly, those who are prone to excessive chattering may distract themselves and others from the task in hand. Other forms of external distraction such as traffic passing a window or conversations being held within earshot may affect the ability to attend to the primary task. As before, any of these factors can interfere to a varying degree depending on the environmental context or overall level of fatigue.

SUSTAINED ATTENTION

Where an individual has the ability to attend to the specified task, the question is then one of the ability to sustain that attention over time. Can attention be sustained longer in certain circumstances? Is it simply a factor of time? Is the period of attention limited to less than that required to complete most tasks or can several tasks be attempted before the attention wanes? If rest periods are allowed, can attention be re-established within the same day?

ALTERNATING OR DIVIDED ATTENTION

Much of what we are all required to do in daily living involves the ability to perform or monitor two activities at the same time, either by switching attention between them until either or both are complete or by splitting our attention between more than one task sufficiently to monitor performance or identify the point at which it is appropriate to attend more consciously to the task, activity or event.

While it may sometimes be difficult to say whether a specific activity requires skills of divided or alternating attention, it is clear that multitasking is required in the home, for example when preparing a meal, and in many lines of work, for example taking minutes and participating in a meeting. It is therefore essential that assessment of attention includes some sort of simulation of such events.

A recent step forward in the quantification of this and many of the other aspects of attention described here has been the publication of the Test of Everyday Attention (Robertson et al 1994), which consists of several sub tests aimed at identifying specific deficits and levels of deficit. These include tasks such as listening for specific lottery numbers on a 10-minute tape and counting a set of auditory tones while ignoring another set.

The results of this standardized test taken together with others, such as the Trail Making Test for Adults (Reitan 1958), and with the observations of multiple informants over a variety of functional circumstances, allow for fairly confident interpretation of an individual's functional attention skills and deficits.

INFORMATION PROCESSING

Another defining factor underpinning performance in general is that of speed of information processing. Put in simple terms, it is necessary to keep up with the speed at which information is normally presented, understanding and interpreting as the event or interaction proceeds, in order to contribute or respond in a meaningful way.

The complexity of how capacity for information relates to memory and other facets of cognition is a subject for debate, but in functional terms those who describe difficulties in dealing with information at speed frequently also complain of becoming 'full up' after relatively short periods of concentration, especially if dealing with new, complex or challenging issues.

Where deficits are fairly severe, reduced speed of processing is clearly detectable within a clinical interaction. A number of aspects of information processing have been targeted within a variety of psychometric tests, and inferences may be drawn from observed performance or time taken in the course of others. Some of the tests that may be referred to by colleagues in this context are the Paced Auditory and Serial Addition Test (PASAT) (Gronwall 1997), the Speed and Capacity of Language Processing (SCOLP) (Baddeley et al 1992) and the Trail Making Test referred to above (Reitan 1958).

LANGUAGE AND COMMUNICATION

The ability to understand and use language and other forms of communication is central to the relationship between the individual and the external environment. Effective communication allows the individual to make sense of external events and to give expression to personal thoughts. Conversely, failure of communication can lead to misunderstanding and to restrictions in the individual's ability to influence the environment around them. Difficulties in these areas have obvious implications for the rehabilitation process.

Successful human communication is a complex and highly skilled interactive process that is, in common with other human functions, not a distinct entity, but is interrelated with other skills and abilities such as motor performance and cognition. The ease with which communication is achieved is also, like other functions, dependent upon the integrity of sensory receptors and their neural connections, and in particular on the auditory and visual systems.

As with the other core skills as described within this approach (see Fig. 5.4), the report of findings on assessment of language and communication skills needs to be interpreted in conjunction with knowledge of the integrity of factors upon which it depends or with which it has a functional relationship. Under each of the proposed subheadings, therefore, it may be necessary to acknowledge specific influencing factors either directly or by reference to detail elsewhere in the full report. The subheadings are in essence a convenient checklist of the primary building blocks upon which successful communication is based and under which significant assessment findings can be summarized.

Assessment of language and speech production is most commonly carried out by speech and language therapists (speech pathologists), but in some instances aspects of the formal assessment may be undertaken by psychologists. However, beyond pure language skills, the assessment of functional communication will benefit from contributions from a variety of observers (Body & Parker 1999).

Indeed, while acknowledging the need to establish the individual's ability level in terms of basic understanding and grammatical construction,

Attention and concentration
Sensation and sensory processing
Motor performance
Language and communication
Memory and learning

Figure 5.4   Core skills

the focus of assessment of communication skills following TBI has shifted away from tests of aphasia, more commonly associated with disability following stroke, and towards the development of functional assessment protocols that are sensitive to the types of functional communication failure more frequently encountered after TBI (Hartley 1990, 1995, McDonald & Pearce 1995).

MOTOR SPEECH

The speed, fluency, intelligibility and emotional qualities of speech may be affected by difficulties of physical production and may be associated with difficulties of mastication and swallowing. The difficulty may be one of absent (anarthric) or impaired (dysarthric) motor performance of the muscles of speech production, inadequate breath support, or other mechanical factors affecting vocalization such as paralysis of the vocal cords.

While dysarthric symptoms are commonly found in the presence of other motor disturbance, more rarely the source of poor or absent vocalization may be speech dyspraxia where there is an inability to articulate appropriately to produce speech although there is no primary neuromuscular weakness. The physical components and background conditions for speech production have been described and may be formally rated via the Frenchay Dysarthria Assessment (Enderby 1983).

VERBAL LANGUAGE

There are many factors influencing the scope and depth of formal assessment that may be carried out to inform the content of this section, which in essence is concerned with the individual's ability to understand fully the spoken word and to be able to use a normal range of vocabulary. There is a range of standardized tests of language skills but they are not commonly used in acute or even subacute TBI provision.

The rationale for using standardized assessments would be to be able to state categorically that basic language skills (of understanding and of expression) are intact or to identify a specific deficit or group of deficits. However, failure to perform well on a test of language may result from other cognitive deficits, for example of attention or orientation, and it is particularly difficult in the early period after TBI to identify the primary reason for the poor performance. Therefore, unless it is necessary to demonstrate that communication is ineffective, it is unlikely to be worthwhile to carry out this type of formal assessment. In addition, if the person to be assessed is agitated or easily aroused, the testing procedure may in itself be detrimental.

Beyond the early stages of recovery, when the individual is considered to be oriented and aware, the influence of other cognitive factors still has to be taken into account in interpreting assessment data. For example, even when basic skills are apparently intact, the individual's ability to use the basic skills in real life must also form part of the global assessment. Thus, the person may perform satisfactorily in a quiet test room but be unable to function where there are competing visual or auditory stimuli, as in a hospital television room or when the children are at play in the home.

These factors and other functional issues will be considered further under the heading of Integration and Organization.

Formal language assessments, such as the Test for Reception of Grammar (TROG) (Bishop 1989) or the Psycholinguistic Assessments of Language Processing in Aphasia (PALPA) (Kay et al 1992), may be used (in full or part) in specific circumstances, and colleagues may use other assessment strategies to examine combined language–cognitive performance, such as tests of verbal fluency, the ability to follow instructions on a real task or to interpret or reiterate information given in a variety of formats.

One of the main errors of health professionals who are not language specialists is the assumption that individuals have good understanding of language when their responses may have been routine or contextually based. Communication is more than language, and understanding may be gained from gesture, facial or vocal characteristics or from environmental cues. And, while an individual's understanding may be sufficient to allow communication of simple ideas or by way of closed (yes/no) questions, they may struggle to follow more complex language.

Thus the skilled observation or informal interview undertaken by the language specialist will be sensitive to compensatory strategies being used in communication, and hypotheses relating to the level of understanding can then be tested by administering a test or subsection of a test at the appropriate level.

INTERACTIVE SKILLS

The assessment of interactive skills (i.e. conversational skills and non-verbal communication) fits well within an integrated assessment approach. Speech and language therapists have the opportunity to observe interactions between the individual being assessed and others, and rich data can also be gathered from the observational report of other team members, based on a wide variety of interactions.

As well as enlisting the observational skills of other health professionals, much information can be obtained from the report of family and friends who observe conversation and social interaction on a daily basis. Information gained from interview or questionnaire can be used to inform the content of the assessment if gathered in advance, or alternatively to test hypotheses by asking probing questions in order to develop a clear overview of conversational behaviour including the contexts within which problems become apparent.

A number of observational rating scales have been developed to allow component analysis of interactive skills. These scales have developed from work in the field of pragmatics (the study of language use in natural contexts) and from discourse analysis (a linguistic approach to analysing and describing language use). The content of some scales is wide and includes such things as clarity of expression, social style, logical content and general participation within conversation (Linscott et al 1996), while others are highly focused such as the Checklist for Listening Behaviours (Hartley 1995).

While these detailed scales have been developed for use by knowledgeable observers, a few global questions regarding the success and comfort of the interactions between the person being assessed and each individual team member can also be incorporated into an observational checklist (Fig. 5.5). The use of multiple informants in the assessment of areas that might be regarded as being based on subjective opinion allows more confident interpretation of the observations than if the assessment was based only on the interaction with a single therapist.

The use of multiple observations can also help begin to identify the context within which vulnerable skills may begin to break down. For example, listening skills may be influenced by the amount of structure imposed on the session, the number of conversational partners or the anxiety level. Thus, someone may be described as having poor listening skills within a session at the beginning of 2 days of assessment but may subsequently be rated by other team members as listening and interacting appropriately. If it can be established that the poor performance was a function of their initial anxiety, a similar performance may be anticipated in other new situations.

Inappropriate or unusual non-verbal behaviours can result from a wide variety of sources; poor eye contact may indicate low mood but may also have developed from strategies to avoid diploplia; failure to observe normal limits of personal space may indicate a degree of disinhibition but, equally, may be the result of a visuoperceptual deficit. There is a clear need to cross reference findings such as these with those of other parts of the assessment before coming to conclusions about their source and, ultimately, about potential interventions.

LITERACY

Finally, in relation to core communication skills there is the question of reading and writing ability. Is the written word recognized and understood, and can thoughts and opinions be freely expressed in writing?

As these skills are complex and functionally interrelated to a number of physical and cognitive dimensions, they potentially may require extensive

OBSERVATIONAL CHECKLIST

Name:

Date:

Interviewer:

	Yes	No	Not observed
Was C aware of errors?	☐	☐	☐
Did C correct errors?	☐	☐	☐
Did C generate ideas/goals appropriately?	☐	☐	☐
Did C plan tasks appropriately?	☐	☐	☐
Did C engage and disengage attention appropriately?	☐	☐	☐
Did C concentrate throughout the session?	☐	☐	☐
Could C deal with more than one thing at once?	☐	☐	☐
Was C distracted by internal/ external stimuli?	☐	☐	☐
Was C's information processing ability reduced?	☐	☐	☐
Did C interact appropriately?	☐	☐	☐
Did C show any strong emotion?	☐	☐	☐
Did C participate fully in session?	☐	☐	☐

Figure 5.5 Staff observational checklist

assessment to define specific difficulties. However, an initial general screen of skills can be obtained via self and carer report of preinjury and present reading habits, by observing the ability to follow written instructions, by including the completion of a simple questionnaire within the assessment process, and by testing everyday functional reading skills at the appropriate level using, for example the newspaper that the individual would usually buy.

MEMORY AND LEARNING

The psychology of memory and learning has been a focus of investigation for many years, and over that period a variety of models, theories and categorizations has been proposed (and some discarded), based on the level of knowledge at the time. Our present understanding of human memory systems emanates initially from laboratory-based studies, but more recently from investigations targeted at gaining knowledge of the mechanisms that underpin memory and learning in real-life functional situations.

This process is still ongoing but memory is clearly regarded as having a pivotal role in learning and functional performance. Lezak (1995, p. 27), in her highly respected textbook on neuropsychological assessment, states:

Central to all cognitive functions and probably to all that is characteristically human in a person's behaviour is the capacity for memory and learning ... Severely impaired memory isolates patients from emotionally or practically meaningful contact with the world around them and deprives them of a sense of personal continuity, rendering them passive and helplessly dependent. Mildly to moderately impaired memory has a disorientating effect.

Functional memory is, then, of great importance, and awareness of the limitations of an individual's memory function must be key knowledge upon which to base all our interactions with that person. We will look at the practical implications of this in Chapter 9.

Memory function is complex but has functionally recognizable subcomponents. The approach to summarizing performance and the headings suggested below are, in the wider context, simplistic. However, they are designed to allow the presentation of assessment findings in such a way as to indicate severity, primary areas of deficit, and performance in terms of functionally recognizable components. While the approach to assessment reporting involves the apparent simplification of complex issues, and although it is not possible to explore this subject fully within the context of this book, there are some basic facts and concepts that are worthy of emphasis.

The fact that memory is not a unitary system means that different deficit profiles can ensue. Thus, evidence of good performance in one area does not imply a fully functioning system. It is of particular note to physiotherapists that while some aspects of motor learning can take place at an implicit level, for example by repetitive experience without explicit recall of each individual experience, this does not mean that the person who demonstrates physical progress within a treatment session will be able to recall verbal instructions to practise an exercise or perform a physical task in a specific way. Equally, while a person may recall an event in general, for example being aware of having been to a treatment session before, they may not recall any of the detail of that event or their recall may be patchy or inaccurate.

We will explore the implications for these types of dysfunction in Chapter 9, but they are included here to illustrate the need for physiotherapists to access and understand the detail of each individual's memory function.

The information to be presented under each heading is synthesized from a variety of sources, depending on the time following injury and the level of recovery of the individual at the time of assessment. As well as formal testing, valuable information can be obtained from existing clinical notes (especially for the evaluation of retrograde and post-traumatic amnesia), from carer and self-report, and via performance on set practical tasks (especially in relation to everyday functional memory). Relevant practical tasks can be incorporated into the assessment process, for example asking the individual to bring sports shorts to facilitate the physical assessment or testing specific recall of a previous session such as their choice when asked to plan a snack or meal.

Many standardized tests are used in the assessment of memory function, some of which are set within full neuropsychological test batteries and some of which are designed to stand alone. The overall conclusion with regard to an individual's memory skills will be based on their performance on many tests of memory and other associated cognitive skills. Each test or subtest examines different aspects of memory function, and a full picture of functional performance and the likely underlying factors can be gleaned only by thorough investigation.

POST-TRAUMATIC AMNESIA

As already discussed, the period of post-traumatic amnesia (PTA) is a strong indicator of the severity of the initial injury. During the period of emergence from deep coma, this may be assessed directly (see Ch. 2). However, this is not established practice and retrospective assessment is usually required. Self-report of primary postinjury memories may be influenced by other cognitive dysfunction such as confabulation or by having been told of events by family or friends.

Corroboration of the individual's report of when continuous recall was established can be sought from those who were present during the period of confusion, including family, friends and health professionals. It is therefore useful routinely to request this information in any referral form and within the carer interview. Although the resultant conclusion will be an estimation, the use of multiple informants, as before, increases confidence in the validity of that estimation.

RETROGRADE AMNESIA

There may be absent memories for a period immediately preceding the injury. Typically this period reduces with recovery, but in some cases a substantial part of the immediate preinjury period does not return. Self-report combined with information gathered from others who were involved in the injured person's life during the period concerned can assist in determining the size and significance of this deficit.

AUTOBIOGRAPHICAL MEMORY

It is important to make the distinction between the individual's ability to recollect information, events and people from earlier periods in life and their ability to manipulate, store and retrieve new information. While the loss of autobiographical memory is not a common occurrence following TBI, it is useful to distinguish actively between the two aspects of memory just described. It is also important to identify the minority who do have problems in this area because of the potential impact of such a deficit on the individual and on any proposed rehabilitation programme.

Standardized assessment in this area is a relatively new development (Kopelman et al 1990) and information is most commonly gathered via questionnaire. It is an area of assessment that relies heavily on corroboration of facts. Some individuals may have difficulty in presenting autobiographical information in a chronological way, but this may reflect other cognitive problems such as difficulty in organizing thoughts or sequencing the presentation of material.

PROSPECTIVE MEMORY

Prospective memory is the ability to remember to do things. This is an aspect of everyday functional memory where deficits are likely to be reported or recognized by those who have regular contact with the person being assessed, and is often recognized and reported by individuals who have adequate memory function to remember their failures. Within the newer functional memory tests, such as the Rivermead Behavioural Memory Test (Wilson et al 1985), aspects of prospective memory can be assessed and analysis of performance on specific tasks set up within the assessment process is useful in gaining an impression of current functional ability.

VERBAL MEMORY AND LEARNING

A variety of neuropsychological tests may be used to be able to describe an individual's ability to register, store and recall verbal material. Via this assessment process a variety of influencing factors, such as internal or external distractors, the speed of presentation of information, or the time it takes to retrieve information, as well as the overall ability to learn new information, will be evaluated. Thus it should be possible to describe a profile of how well the person being assessed is able to deal with verbal material.

This ability will vary across the TBI population from a global failure to hold on to any new information to very specific difficulties such as the need for repeated presentation, the need to limit the volume of information presented, the need for time to process the information, or the need for some prompt to facilitate recall. In the presence of deficits specific strategies may also be observed, for example confabulation in the presence of poor recall.

NON-VERBAL MEMORY AND LEARNING

The ability to process and recall non-verbal material may be evaluated in a similar way to that described above to produce the same kind of ability profile.

It is probably worthwhile reiterating the interdependent nature of memory and learning with other cognitive functions, and to emphasize the value of physiotherapists being aware of, and understanding the nature of, an individual's cognitive profile. For example, if someone demonstrates problems with non-verbal learning, it may not be appropriate to ask them to make their own way from ward to department or from waiting area to treatment room without first ensuring that they can learn the route.

INTEGRATION AND ORGANIZATION

Having described abilities and deficits at core skill level, with appropriate reference to the current psychosocial status, consideration then needs to be given to the individual's ability to integrate their preserved abilities to produce meaningful function.

The term 'integration and organization' is used within this approach to global assessment reporting as it allows consideration of all the manifestations of poor integration and organizational ability without the confines of function associated with particular brain locations or conceptualized syndromes. Thus, while much of the functional ability under scrutiny within this section is synonymous with what might be referred to elsewhere as *executive function*, and although disorders of executive function are frequently found in relation to frontal lobe damage, we are not here either restricting ourselves to, or examining all of, frontal lobe function.

Having said that, a basic understanding of the impact of the functional limitations associated with difficulties in integration and organization may be gained with reference to the working definition proposed by Mayer and colleagues (1990, p. 263), who state:

the executive disorder reflects, at least in part, an impaired ability to formulate and maintain intentions and to resolve competing intentions without their resulting in error.

Thus, while individuals may or may not have particular core skill deficits, their functional performance may be limited not by basic ability but by problems in integrating the relevant skills and processes and applying them in an appropriate way. This section attempts to look at the main components of the normal sequence of goal formation, planning and execution of an intended action to identify those aspects that are, and are not, intact.

As in other areas of evaluation where assessment is reliant on comparison with *normal* values, there is a need for caution in the interpretation of observational data, particularly as some of the issues under consideration by their nature may be regarded as personal characteristics or behavioural traits. We all know people who manage their lives via the compilation of endless lists, who like to plan each move and to follow those plans through in sequence. Equally, there are people who are more spontaneous, and indeed chaotic, in their approach.

The important point is that although both of these approaches have a very different emphasis they would, in normal circumstances, produce a successful functional outcome. Therefore, both the component parts, and the cumulative result (the functional outcome), of the approach adopted by the individual being assessed need to be included in the overall analysis, with particular emphasis being given to the functional outcome.

The main factors under consideration are, the ability to:

- Generate and develop realistic goals
- Plan and action activities to achieve identified goals
- Monitor performance during activities, recognizing and acknowledging errors
- Problem-solve to correct errors.

These skills and behaviours can be evaluated by way of formal testing, structured observation and information gathering with regard to both approach and success in real-life activities.

There are, as in the case of other cognitive functions, established psychometric tests that may be administered to inform ability level and approach. A recent addition to assessment in this area has been the Behavioural Assessment of the Dysexecutive Syndrome (BADS) (Wilson et al 1996), which can be administered by trained professionals other than psychologists.

However, it is also useful to assess performance during a life-appropriate activity and to seek information with regard to performance in real situations, so that comparison can be made between findings. Additional information can be gleaned from comparing performance between previously routine activities and more novel activities that require a higher level of immediate attention and problem solving.

Indications of potential difficulties in integration and organization may also come from the analysis of observed or reported negative behaviours.

Case example 5.1   Analysis of Tom's behaviour

Tom's reported problem was general irritability and sudden verbal outbursts, which both Tom and his wife described as a consistent change in his personality.

Questioning revealed three frequent peaks of verbal aggression: in early morning, late afternoon and mid evening. Further discussion also highlighted a childcare–food link, that is, at these times Tom was trying to persuade a child in his care to get on with necessary organizational activities (like getting dressed or undressed, or washing hands) while preparing snacks or drinks that involved directing or monitoring activities in an adjacent room.

The analysis was (as confirmed by Tom) that, because he had on previous occasions forgotten about items on the cooker, he focused his attention on the kitchen activities and resisted other distractions. His interactions with others at these times became terse and abrupt, and this was perceived as irritability. The outbursts usually occurred when a third party (any other family member) tried to enter into conversation with Tom or the child, and especially when the interaction included questions or introduced uncertainty that demanded additional thought or decision on Tom's part.

In terms of core skills assessment, Tom's memory function was only mildly impaired (having difficulty with quantity of information and failing to register information in the presence of distraction). His basic language skills were intact except for a tendency to interpret phrases in a literal way rather than the interpretation found in common everyday usage. However, formal tests did highlight some difficulty in making choices and in making progress in tasks that required the mental manipulation of two ideas at the same time. Thus, while his core deficits appeared minimal, the functional impact in terms of performance anxiety, ineffective communication and behavioural sequelae was significant.

The analysis of the situational behaviour and cross-referencing with formal assessment findings allowed the development of understanding by the professionals and by Tom and his family, which then formed the basis of coping strategies for this specific and other similar situations. This included the decision not to design his physical intervention programme to be based in the family home, except at times when space and privacy, with no external distraction, could be guaranteed.

This link was used to analyse, explain and ultimately reduce a negative behaviour reported by the wife of Tom, who was referred to in Chapter 4 (see Case examples 4.3 and 5.1).

REFERENCES

Baddeley A D, Emslie H, Nimmo-Smith I 1992 The speed and capacity of language-processing test. Thames Valley Test Company, Bury St Edmunds

Bishop D V M 1989 Test for the reception of grammar. 2nd edn. Medical Research Council Applied Psychology Unit, Cambridge

Body R, Parker M 1999 The use of multiple informants in assessment of communication after traumatic brain injury. In: McDonald S, Togher L, Code C (eds) Communication disorders following traumatic brain injury. Psychology Press, Hove, p 147

Enderby P 1983 The Frenchay dysarthria assessment. College Hill Press, San Diego, CA

Goldberg D, Williams P 1988 A user's guide to the general health questionnaire. NFER-Nelson, Windsor, UK

Gronwall D M A 1997 Paced auditory serial-addition task: a measure of recovery from concussion. Perceptual and Motor Skills 44:367–373

Hartley L L 1990 Assessment of functional communication. In: Tupper D E, Cicerone K D (eds) The neuropsychology of everyday life, vol 1: assessment and basic competencies. Kluwer Academic Publishers, Boston, MA, p 125

Hartley L L 1995 Cognitive–communicative abilities following brain injury: a functional approach. Singular Publishing, San Diego, CA

Kay J, Lesser R, Coltheart M 1992 PALPA: psycholinguistic assessments of language processing in aphasia. Lawrence Erlbaum, Hove

Kopelman M, Wilson B, Baddeley A 1990 The autobiographical memory interview. Thames Valley Test Company, Bury St Edmunds

Lezak M D 1995 Neuropsychological assessment, 3rd edn. Oxford University Press, New York

Linscott R J, Knight R G, Godfrey I I P D 1996 The profile of functional impairment in communication (PFIC): a measure of communication impairment for clinical use. Brain Injury 10(6):397–412

McDonald S, Pearce S 1995 The 'dice' game: a new test of pragmatic language skills after closed-head injury. Brain Injury 9(3):255–271

McWilliams S 1991 Affective changes following severe head injury as perceived by patients and relatives. British Journal of Occupational Therapy 54:246–248

Mayer H M, Reed E, Schwartz M F, Montgomery M, Palmer C 1990 Buttering a hot cup of coffee: an approach to the study of errors of action in patients with brain damage. In: Tupper D E, Cicerone K D (eds) The neuropsychology of everyday life: assessment and basic competencies, 1st edn. Kluwer Academic, Norwell, p 259

Reitan R M 1958 Validity of the trail making test as an indicator of organic brain damage. Perceptual and Motor Skills 8:271–276

Robertson I H, Ward T, Ridgeway V, Nimmo-Smith I 1994 The test of everyday attention. Thames Valley Test Company, Bury St Edmunds

Tyerman A, Humphrey M 1984 Changes in self-concept following severe head injury. International Journal of Rehabilitation and Research 7:11 23

Wilson B, Cockburn J, Baddeley A 1985 The Rivermead behavioural memory test. Thames Valley Test Company, Bury St Edmunds

Wilson B, Alderman N, Burgess P W, Emslie H, Evans J J 1996 Behavioural assessment of the dysexecutive syndrome. Thames Valley Test Company, Bury St Edmunds

Zigmond A S, Snaith R P 1983 The Hospital Anxiety and Depression Scale. Acta Psychiatrica Scandinavica 67(6):361–370

6

Sensorimotor assessment

Key Points

- Sensory perception and motor performance are inextricably linked in the process of learning and enacting functional movement, but physiotherapeutic assessment has tended to be more oriented to the motor output area of this cyclical process
- Sensory evaluation should be a clear focus of TBI assessment, although the question of how to undertake a systematic sensory assessment has barely begun to be discussed in the literature; a schematic approach to the assessment and discussion of sensory dysfunction is proposed and described
- Assessment of motor performance in the presence of neuropathology remains as varied as the treatment approaches and therapeutic concepts espoused by individual neurophysiotherapists, but there are some core factors across the majority of approaches to assessment; a pragmatic approach to the reporting of motor performance assessment findings is proposed along with a basic structure of headings and some suggestion of how to shape the process of analysis
- Issues surrounding the assessment of the true level of functional activity conclude the discussion of the information-gathering section of the assessment process

INTRODUCTION

Having described the content and process of information gathering for areas of the global assessment peripheral to the primary focus of the physiotherapist, this chapter now looks at the two specific core skill sections that require detailed analysis by the physiotherapist: sensation and sensory processing, and motor performance. The outline of the global assessment is then completed with reference to actual functional performance as described under the heading of Life skills.

SENSATION AND SENSORY PROCESSING

The ability of each individual to appreciate, analyse, interpret and use sensory information is a multifactorial and complex process. Although effective processing of sensory information is recognized as crucial to the production of skilled movement, the systematic assessment of sensory function remains an underdeveloped area in neurophysiotherapeutic practice.

Given the potential for disruption of sensory perception at any point from primary receptor level through all areas of integration and interpretation, it would seem that the evaluation of sensory systems following traumatic brain injury (TBI) should receive significant attention during assessment. On the other hand, if this argument is followed to its logical conclusion, acknowledging the importance of the primary senses, the peripheral tactile system and the proprioceptive system including the vestibular system, then the scope of potential dysfunction is seen to be very large, and therefore difficult for any single profession to tackle in full in the clinical setting.

There are, however, other reasons why physiotherapists are not always proactive in identifying sensory deficits and why the apparently clear need for comprehensive sensory assessment has not been fully developed in the hospital or clinic. For example, rehabilitative practice in the UK has developed so that within routine clinical practice the interpretative or cognitive aspects of sensation (often called perception) are regarded as the province of the occupational therapist or the psychologist. Thus, the impact of sensory dysfunction on motor performance, and vice versa, has not always been considered, contributing to the continuing false delineation between sensation and action.

Brazzelli & Della Sala (1997) clearly articulate the interrelationship between sensation, cognition and motor function, and highlight the need for collaboration between physiotherapists and neuropsychologists to overcome this functionally unhelpful delineation, for the benefit of the patient. They argue that accurate assessment of the root cause of many motor deficits requires knowledge of cognition, including sensory processing, and conclude that neuropsychology should be taught in the schools of physiotherapy.

Another example of a barrier to holistic assessment is the practice in some areas of the USA where interprofessional delineation is complicated further by differentiating responsibility for aspects of rehabilitation between occupational therapists and physiotherapists in line with predominantly upper limb or ambulatory function.

In addition to these confusions in therapeutic practice, assessment pertaining to the primary senses may traditionally be carried out by a variety of specialist medical practitioners and their technicians. Therefore, perhaps more than in any other domain, team discussion in advance of defining the assessment process with regard to the purpose of, relationship between, and responsibility for sensory testing will prove to be a productive use of time.

Moreover, approaching sensory assessment in this way may also facilitate the development of an attitude to assessment that permits some flexibility in the presently fairly rigid practice of clinicians feeling the need *personally* to gather *all* the assessment information they need to plan their particular specialist intervention.

In summary, then, sensation and sensory processing is a large and complex area. Given the potential for dysfunction at any, or many, levels within the sensory system following TBI, sensory evaluation should be a clear focus within the team assessment. However, a systematic, clear assessment process has yet to be defined for use in clinical practice, and sensory assessment is often tackled in a piecemeal fashion, involving a wide variety of professionals. There is no agreed format for communicating the scope or findings of a clinical sensory evaluation between therapists of the same discipline or across the multidisciplinary team.

A SCHEMATIC APPROACH TO SENSORY ASSESSMENT

To plan an approach to sensory assessment and then communicate which aspects have been assessed and which have not, it may be useful to adopt a schematic model. Such a model is represented diagrammatically in Figure 6.1.

At the basis of this working model, there are the primary sensory receptors and end organs, for example sensory nerve endings, muscle spindles or the vestibular apparatus. Then, linking these with the central nervous system, there are the primary neural links (i.e. the peripheral and cranial nerves), which may transmit directly or may merge with other sensory input along the way. Activity within the central nervous system is summarized as occurring at an initial integrative level, capable of producing a

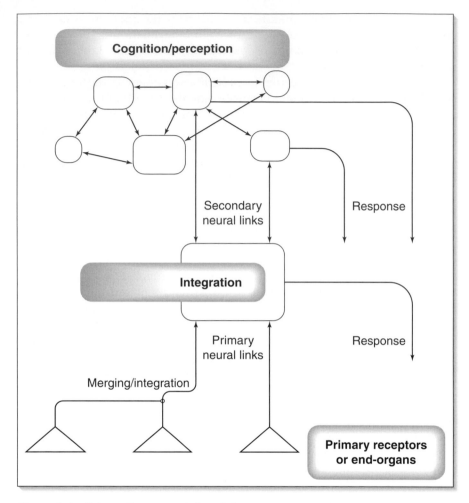

Figure 6.1   Schematic representation of the sensory processing system

direct response and then at a more sophisticated level of integration with additional processed sensory and other stored information.

This simplified overview of sensory processing is suggested as a way of conceptualizing the gross levels of function that should be considered when examining sensory function, to aid assessment planning, interpretation of findings, and as a basis for communicating findings to others. It is important, however, to appreciate that in normal circumstances there is a constant inflow of sensory information and a constant vigilance by the central nervous system in the form of ongoing perception, interpretation and communication with other central structures. Therefore, to be functional, the sensory system has not only to be intact at all the levels described in the model but also has to be able to function within this ongoing multifactorial context.

So, following this schematic approach, assessment needs to consider the primary receptors and their connections and the primary and secondary levels of processing and perception. In addition, because of the prevalence of reduced speed of information processing in this population, sensory assessment should also include consideration of the speed of response to sensory stimulation. Finally, given the interrelationships between specific sensory systems, and with particular reference to the visual, vestibular and neck proprioceptive systems, observation and enquiry regarding evidence of sensory mismatch or apparent conflict should also be included.

Additional considerations in assessment and report design

By virtue of all the subsystems that could conceivably be examined, and the potentially time-consuming nature of this activity, it may be possible, even with the resources of a full team, to perform only a screening assessment at initial contact. In addition, given the subjective nature of much of the data to be gathered, and the fact that the validity of the subjective assessment is interdependent with aspects such as level of arousal, attention and communication, definitive assessment of sensory function may be possible only beyond the acute period, towards the later stages of recovery. It is important, therefore, to be cautious in recording that an individual is sensorially intact in advance of some level of definitive testing at a time when subjective report may be regarded as reliable.

Before designing the assessment protocol, and again before attempting to document a synthesis of the clinical and laboratory findings, it is useful to acknowledge coexisting factors that influence the perception and/or subjective report of sensation. In terms of interpreting and reporting findings, this may mean cross-referencing with other sections of the assessment, for example acknowledging the influence of other cognitive problems as detailed above or other physical influences, such as a motor control problem producing diplopia or the presence of splints or casts preventing full examination.

PROCEDURE

While recognizing that this approach to assessment is far removed from an exact science, it is suggested that, given the complexity of the sensory system, an adequate screen should target each subsystem, where possible, at both end organ and integration–perception levels. The main objectives of this type of screening are:

- To identify or exclude peripheral dysfunction
- To highlight the need for further assessment either within the team or via referral to other specialized practitioner(s)
- To begin to identify and document sensory dysfunction requiring focused intervention or likely to impact on the design or delivery of wider planned intervention.

SUBJECTIVE REPORT OF SYMPTOMS AND FUNCTIONAL DIFFICULTIES

Where the individual is able to communicate or if there is other reliable evidence of their discomfort or complaints over the recent time period, it is useful to start the process of information gathering from their subjective report of symptoms and functional difficulties. A checklist to standardize the enquiry around physical complaints will aid the efficiency and inclusiveness of the enquiry.

Sensory perception, including pain, is a subjective and personal experience (Sim & Waterfield 1997, Sluka & Rees 1997) and it is important to try to ensure a clear understanding of what the individual means by the descriptive vocabulary they use. It is also important for the assessor not to assign their own description without ascertaining its appropriateness.

The enquiry should identify both preinjury deficits and changes since the time of injury and should cover:

- The senses of smell and taste: perception (is it there at all), discrimination (can all differentiations be made)
- Vision: any form of visual degradation, what form it takes and when or how it occurs; any sensitivities (to light, when fatigued, during headache, when reading), visual illusions, changes in perception of the environment
- Hearing: degradation, sensitivities (to what, in what context and what is the effect)
- Subjective awareness of peripheral sensory changes (absence, altered, noxious)
- Pain (quality, site, frequency, provoking factors, associations)
- Dizziness, sensations of disorientation or disassociation, nausea, feelings of imbalance (quality, frequency, provoking factors, associations)

ASSESSMENT OF PRIMARY SENSORY FUNCTION

It is difficult to test the function of peripheral end organs in isolation, especially in the clinical setting, since in most cases examination is also dependent on the integrity of the associated peripheral or cranial nerves, and on their central connections. However, as part of a wider approach and by a process of elimination, findings of assessment focused towards the integrity of the peripheral apparatus will contribute to the identification of the deficit level.

Using documented information

Records of previous clinical assessments or specialist laboratory investigations may be available, for example the cranial nerve examination carried out during the medical evaluation, the results of visual field tests, audiological examination or laboratory tests of peripheral vestibular function. Where such information is not available, or if it is appropriate to reassess to establish the stability or otherwise of some deficits, the team may decide specifically to screen particular modalities.

Screening selected modalities

It may be appropriate, for example, to test the sense of smell using bottled, prepared aromas or common household substances as part of a risk assessment. If there is a question about an individual's ability to respond to auditory stimuli, a simple test of hearing using a tuning fork may be undertaken to help determine the need for full audiological assessment.

A standard prerequisite of the wider sensory examination is the assessment of oculomotor function and visual acuity. For example, observations can be made of resting eye positions, the range and quality of horizontal, vertical, diagonal and circular eye movements, and reported changes in the quality of vision during testing can also be recorded.

It is also important to check the ability to move visual attention from one focal object to another elsewhere in the visual field in a timely and efficient way. Although the ability to move visual attention quickly, accurately and selectively is controlled by central structures, it is essential to eliminate this type of central dysfunction as the source of apparent sensory visual dysfunction.

In terms of visual acuity, this can be screened using a Snellen chart, wearing prescribed glasses if appropriate, to establish a basic ability to see the detail of visual information or highlight the need for specialist visual assessment.

Tactile and proprioceptive sensation

A variety of materials and procedures has been suggested in attempts to standardize assessment of limb tactile and proprioceptive sensation. Much of this work has been developed with regard to assessing individual modalities in the field of peripheral nerve damage and the more complex systems are presently most applicable for use in evaluation of specific treatments in the research context (for a review see Van Deusen & Foss 1997).

A great deal of basic work remains to be done in terms of standardization of clinical practice (Winward et al 1998) and in achieving acceptable levels of inter-rater reliability (Lincoln et al 1991), so that clinical assessment most relevant to designing treatments and/or predicting outcome can then be developed. Carey and colleagues (1996, 1997) have already begun to address some of these issues within the stroke population, incorporating the need to test interpretative dysfunction in this client group as dictated by the central nature of the sensory lesions they experience and thus, if we refer to our schematic model, testing at the higher level of integration of sensory information.

In the same way, while it may be appropriate to test individual modalities thoroughly in isolated body parts, for example when concomitant peripheral nerve or spinal injury is suspected, it is unlikely to be feasible and probably of little functional value to carry out a whole-body in-depth assessment as routine following TBI. It is therefore important to consider carefully what aspects of testing to include in a screening of tactile and proprioceptive sensation and also to be aware of the limitations on interpretation imposed by the chosen procedure.

For example, in some areas it is common practice to assume integrity of joint position and movement sense in the upper limb if accurate responses are obtained on testing the finger joints. This may a dangerous assumption given the research evidence suggesting that the joints of the fingers and toes differ from larger proximal joints in the percentage contribution of pressure and tactile sensation in the assessment of joint position and movement (Clarke et al 1979, 1985).

We should also be aware that, in testing awareness of joint position and motion by moving the body part for the individual, we are removing a normally powerful source of proprioceptive information that emanates from the muscles activated during the process of voluntary movement (Gandevia et al 1992). It may be necessary, where active movement is absent, for the assessor to move the body part to assess gross proprioceptive awareness, but a more accurate predictor of functional proprioceptive awareness will be gained by assessing via active movement.

One further consideration in the design of a tactile and proprioceptive screen for reasons of safety is the need to identify any localized abnormalities in the threshold of pain appreciation.

Dizziness

Finally in relation to the contribution of peripheral factors to sensory dysfunction, we need to consider the question of dizziness and disorientation. As a wider concept, this area is at present poorly understood and only sparsely documented in the TBI literature. There are multiple potential sources of dizziness and disorientation after TBI and we will go on to consider some of these in terms of the integration and processing of sensory information.

Peripheral vestibular dysfunction is an accepted primary source of dizziness following TBI, with a reported incidence of between 30% and 65% (Shumway-Cook 1994), and dizziness of central (brain) origin is also well recognized (Shepard & Teilan 1996). There is also evidence to suggest that dizziness may emanate from visual dysfunction (Bronstein 1995) and from dysfunction of the cervical spine (Karlberg 1995).

Clinical recognition of dizziness and the identification of provoking factors via interview and physical assessment are possible to some degree, but accurate attribution of the primary source is often more difficult, especially where there is limited access to a neuro-otological or neuro-ophthalmological opinion. Where these are available, the combination of specialist medical assessment, laboratory studies carried out by vestibular scientists and orthoptic evaluation is invaluable in confirming or excluding peripheral vestibular sources of dizziness and in highlighting potential additional or alternative sources.

ASSESSMENT OF INTEGRATIVE SENSORY FUNCTION

When the peripheral aspects of a sensory subsystem appear intact, or when self-report or structured observation has highlighted the possibility of functional failure that is not explained by the peripheral screen, further consideration of central dysfunction is indicated. The schematic model separates this type of dysfunction into problems of either integration or interpretation. In this context, problems of integration would be best described as limitations in the speed or volume of sensory information that can be processed effectively.

Thus, we are not talking about the cognitive aspects of sensation, such as perception, or the effective interpretation and application of sensory information that results in appropriate action, but what might be regarded as the mechanics of processing all the relevant sensory information within the appropriate temporal constraints. Thus, while testing proprioception at joint level an individual may be able to describe the position of the joint with reasonable accuracy, when tested at multi-joint level, say involving a whole limb, their ability is more obviously dysfunctional.

A functional example of the effects of this type of disorder would be when someone with apparently intact peripheral sensation, visual functioning and vestibular function (as tested independently) cannot successfully respond to a sudden change in their sensory environment. Such an individual may well deal with the majority of physical demands but at the same time report a tendency to overbalance and/or excessive fatigue when pursuing a normal range of physical activities.

Another aspect of dysfunction at the level of integrating sensory information which needs to be examined in the course of the assessment is that which presents as nausea or dizziness or is sometimes reported as feelings of disassociation, imbalance or unsteadiness. All these noxious sensations are thought to result from a variety of forms of sensory mismatch or sensory conflict involving the very closely related and functionally interdependent vestibular, visual and proprioceptive systems.

The three systems contribute to the overall knowledge of whether one is in equilibrium with one's environment and if one's body parts are appropriately oriented for the effective prosecution of the task in hand. In normal function, information from all these systems is cross-referenced and, through experience (of successful motor behaviour), agreement is learned and subsequently recognized as normal (Carpenter 1996). Incoming signals are continually checked for agreement, and minor adjustments or recalibrations are made in the presence of consistent error signals (Zee 1994).

The deduced theory of sensory conflict and the error signals that are perceived as the noxious sensation have been accepted as part of the basis for the symptoms of motion sickness and other similar *naturally occurring* phenomenon, and also as an explanation for the dizziness associated with acquired peripheral vestibular function (Curthoys & Baloh 1995). It also appears to be a credible explanation for the variety of subjective negative sensations reported by individuals who have dysfunctional visual systems or neck proprioceptive systems or central deficits that impact on the efficiency of the normal cross-referencing, selective processing or recalibrating processes (Berman & Fredrickson 1978).

Often such feelings are transient in nature and diminish as the new information, regularly presented, is recognized and given normal status via the process of recalibration. However, where the noxious sensations are avoided or where the central mechanisms normally responsible for the calibrating process are themselves dysfunctional, protracted difficulties may be experienced. Therefore, if an individual consistently reports sensations of dizziness, disorientation, imbalance or a fear of activity, consideration should be given to a sensory source and assessment should not be limited to evaluation of the peripheral vestibular system.

The importance of screening the motor function of the visual system has already been mentioned and the efficiency of the link between the vestibular and visual systems can be checked by looking at vestibulo-ocular reflex (VOR) function. While clinical VOR tests are relatively straightforward to apply, the rationale behind them and the interpretation of findings, especially when diffuse brain injury is present, are more complex. Interested practitioners are referred to two excellent textbooks (Herdman 1994, Shepard & Teilan 1996) for further background reading.

Individuals who report disorientation or fatigue in particular circumstances or environments may be sensitive to particular types of sensory information such as bright or ultraviolet lights or vibrant patterns. Careful enquiry can help build a picture of what constitutes the stressful situation. For those who wish to explore the question of visual stress in more depth, the book *Visual stress* (Wilkins 1995) is recommended.

Clinical experience has also highlighted a link between neck pathology (rarely involving bony injury) and various reports of disequilibrium, abnormal sensations or, in some cases, habitual avoidance of physical activity. This clinically observed link is not confined to TBI and has been documented following whiplash and other cervical spine pathology (Karlberg 1995); it has also been described in experimental research (de Jong et al 1976). Thus, the observed and reported response to active head movements, and probably to trunk rotation with the head held static, should be included in the screening assessment.

Specific tests of sensory integration as related to balance function have been developed for use in the clinic (Shumway-Cook & Horak 1986) and with the aid of computerized equipment (Nashner 1993, Voorhees 1989, 1990). These may be useful in helping define functional habits, including compensatory strategies, and may also aid treatment planning.

To summarize, there is a level of sensory processing beyond peripheral function and separate from other more readily recognized 'higher' sensory functions that may cause functional difficulties for individuals after TBI. Sensory assessment needs to include testing of the individual's reaction to high-speed and high-volume sensory stimuli and a search for the source of reported or observed symptoms of sensory conflict or suboptimal motor performance.

SENSORY PERCEPTION

Standardized assessments of specific aspects of sensory perception have been developed and are used routinely by neuropsychologists, to a lesser degree by occupational therapists and, in relation to auditory perception, by speech and language therapists. Some tests focus on one specific aspect and others screen for a number of functions. Again, the potential scope of testing prohibits definitive testing during one or even two assessment sessions, so the objectives of the initial screening assessment should be agreed in advance.

One or two multifaceted tests may be used to identify any areas of concern which may subsequently be examined further. However, it is also useful to remember that, while some problems may well be clearly identified during testing, the nature of the tests, with their bias towards visuospatial deficits, may not identify all functional problems. This caution should also be applied when considering the perceptual aspects, or individual subjective interpretation, of those dysfunctional integrative and processing elements of sensory function discussed above.

In addition, misperceived tactile or kinaesthetic sensations giving rise to descriptions of abnormal awareness of certain body parts or misperceived relationship between body and environment should also be considered as the source of aberrant behaviour. Physiotherapists may be in the best position to link these two aspects via their observation of motor behaviour during the assessment process.

Essentially, while aspects of perception, particularly visual perception, are understood and the cerebral source of dysfunction may be known, there is no complete theory of perception that allows us to develop a strategic assessment. Thus, a combination of tests of discrete perceptual functions and other basic components thought to underpin multiple functional activities, along with skilled observations of the individual tackling real functional activities, will be required to gain a holistic picture of the integrity of the individual's perceptual skills.

MOTOR PERFORMANCE

The assessment or evaluation of motor performance in a clinical setting is undoubtedly the primary province of the physiotherapist. However, clinical practice within the wider field of neurological physiotherapy is not consistent across the profession in terms of the treatment approach used and assessment processes, even within treatment approaches, are not yet standardized.

Over the past 25 years much work has gone into developing a variety of measures in an attempt to standardize assessment practices (e.g. Ashburn & members of the Motor Club 1982, Lincoln & Leadbitter 1979) and to provide a structure for the measurement of treatment outcomes (e.g. Mawson 1993). However, the issues surrounding the divergence of theoretical treatment approaches and the cultural propensity within the profession to prioritize time towards hands-on therapy rather than detailed written records, combined with a number of other factors, have worked against the development of a globally acceptable assessment protocol for acquired neuropathology.

These wider issues are discussed in detail in relation to the application of neurophysiotherapeutic principles in Chapter 8 but the resultant situation is that, at present, there remains a variety of treatment approaches, an even greater variety of assessment protocols, and only limited use of objective measures.

However, for the purposes of reporting the assessment of motor performance after TBI in the same level of detail as the other core skills referred to in this consideration of global assessment needs, it is suggested that findings, from whatever source(s), should be synthesized and presented under a number of standard subheadings. The scope of the assessment of motor performance and the subheadings used will vary depending on the functional level of the individual being assessed, and to some extent will also be determined by the time since injury at which the assessment takes place.

The standard assessment report headings given are suggested as being core in that they reflect the main functional starting positions (sitting and standing) and the starting point for mobile function (walking). In this approach detailed report of motor performance in lying is not automatically included and would be inserted only when the motor behaviours observed in the course of the assessment are such that they contribute substantially to the understanding of the whole motor performance picture. This would be the case, for example, if a modified lying position was found to be a primary functional position, as in the minimally responsive or severely physically restricted individual. In these circumstances a description of ability in this maximally supportive position is likely to form the majority of the report on motor performance.

Similarly it may be informative to note difficulties of tolerating weight-bearing in particular positions, as is often found with particular sensory deficits, or notable responses, such as increased alertness, when placed in positions not achievable through the individual's own effort.

At the other end of the performance spectrum it should be remembered that, within this approach to assessment report structure, task-related functional ability is covered elsewhere (see Life skills below), and that this section on motor performance represents a breakdown only of the background baseline physical limitations and abilities upon which an indeterminate number of physical functions are based.

The intent, as in other sections, is that related observations are brought together and summarized under each of the headings to give the reader a clear picture of the issues at hand. Therefore, before summarizing the findings for an external audience, the physiotherapist can follow any variety of assessment approaches, with or without objective measures, and record the detailed findings in the therapeutic notes. Subsequently, by way of the process of drawing together and synthesizing all the recorded findings, interpreting them in the context of the broader assessment and presenting them in a manner that is comprehensible to other healthcare professionals, the physiotherapist should become more aware of the relative importance of the raw assessment findings, making the development of functionally relevant treatment goals a relatively simple process.

TOWARDS A FLEXIBLE MODEL OF ASSESSMENT

Within each of the major approaches to neurophysiotherapeutic intervention, no matter what their theoretical basis, the concept of assessment to identify variation from the normal has been employed. Following the assessment and identification of the components of movement that are thought to be less than optimal, intervention in the first instance is then commonly targeted at remediation. However, both the focus of the intervention and the strategy and methods used will differ across treatment approaches. For example, one therapist may attend to what is thought to be an underlying problem, such as abnormal muscle tone or soft tissue adaptation, while another may choose to use activities to improve the performance of the movement itself, such as supervised and critiqued practice of reaching for an everyday object, or the rehearsal of specific aspects of gait.

However, although the ultimate diagnosis of the *key* underlying problem, and therefore the relevant treatment strategy, may not yet be consensual, there are points of agreement in the process of assessment common to most approaches. These are based on core physiotherapeutic knowledge of the biomechanics and neural control of posture, balance and movement, and include the observation of:

- The ability to achieve and maintain the major functional starting positions (postural control, equilibrium)
- The ability to enact independent functional motor activities from the positional base (skilled action)
- The ability to move between different positions (gross functional movement)
- The ease with which more complex functional movements, such as those involving upper limb or head movement during ambulation, can be attempted or achieved (automatic execution and adaptation of sophisticated functional movement).

All these observations involve a combination of rating the achievement of a motor goal and an assessment of the quality of action used in achieving the goal. Where the goal is not achieved, or when the action is assessed as being abnormal or inefficient, the suboptimal performance is then attributed to a variety of factors and the factors that are emphasized will be dependent on the theoretical basis of the therapist's clinical practice.

Much of the content of the assessment and outcome scales developed for use within neurophysiotherapeutic practice attempt to standardize such an observational approach, although they have adopted varying degrees of emphasis on detail or level of measurement. The main problem in recommending the use of one standard assessment for use in TBI is that most published scales have been designed for, and validated for use with, the stroke population, presuming a degree of normality on the so-called unaffected side.

The assessment overview presented in this section, and indeed throughout this chapter, results from an endeavour to develop an appropriate standardized assessment of motor performance after TBI which began a decade ago and, although such a physical assessment was derived from first principles and has been tested to some degree and developed through clinical use, it has not being fully validated. I am sure there are other schedules in clinical use that suffer from the same inadequacies of development but the issue is that they, like my own, are not in the public domain, available for others to use or develop.

This is something that the global profession needs to address and we could begin by recognizing the complexity of the philosophical, knowledge-base and practical reasons why assessment standards and processes for TBI have apparently failed to be produced and evaluated. As this is a complex and unresolved issue, and because it is linked inextricably with the design and delivery of interventions, this will be discussed in Chapter 8.

However, from the experience of trying to develop an adequate assessment I presently hold two beliefs. The first is that it is impossible to develop a *single* assessment schedule that will cover all patients with TBI, and which is also feasible to use within routine clinical practice. The second is that while our understanding of the detail of the neural control of movement, especially in the presence of pathology, is continually changing and developing it is probably not realistic to claim to measure things such as spasticity, of which we do not have a full understanding.

My conclusion is that we should focus on developing a variety of component assessments that may be used discretely or in a variety of combinations, as appropriate to the level of functioning or the potential scope of intervention, and that we should focus, for the present at least, on aspects where we can hope to achieve some level of interobserver reliability in the clinical setting.

Whatever objective measures we develop or adapt, and while we still lack consensus on what to use, we still have to be able to synthesize our findings to understand how they interrelate and to make them understandable to others. It is the structure of this process that is outlined throughout the rest of this section.

Bases and principles of reporting

The approach to assessment reporting outlined here is developed from the learning described above and presumes core knowledge of human posture and movement analysis. It attempts to use language that is understandable to any physiotherapist, no matter what philosophical approach to treatment they may follow. It focuses on the observable, but offers the opportunity for the therapist to formulate links between various observations and to offer opinion on the causal factors. Thus, while the structural approach to reporting has an apparently strong biomechanical emphasis, this should be regarded more as a baseline frame of reference than an exclusion of neurophysiological or neuropathological factors.

As well as describing the relationship between what is biomechanically *normal* (where this is known) and the individual patient's performance, the factors contributing to performance level, whether they be skeletal restriction, a failure to recruit adequate activity in certain muscle groups, apparent overactivity within other muscle groups or some overarching movement disorder such as an involuntary tremor, can easily be added to the description.

The emphasis is on presenting an adequate picture of performance and dysfunction in enough detail and with sufficient clarity of language that it may be understood by all health professionals. It presumes that the physiotherapist will be skilled enough to bring together the data from observations and measurement and to interpret how they interact to effect the functional performance as described. The report should not, therefore, include lists of measurements without any indication of their functional impact and it should, when applicable, include a description of how certain dysfunctions observed in a specific position link with others described within the section.

The progression through major functional starting positions reflects and applies the structured observation common to most approaches to intervention already described (see Table 6.1 for a review). The core functional positions are considered first and then special consideration is given to the assessment of individuals at both ends of the spectrum of functional performance: the minimally active and those performing at a high level.

Factors influencing motor performance

Motor performance is not a discrete act and can obviously be influenced by a number of intrinsic and extrinsic factors. When reporting assessment

Table 6.1 Components of motor performance common to the assessment process across therapeutic approaches

Observations	Level of performance
Ability to achieve and maintain the major functional starting positions	Postural control, equilibrium
Ability to enact independent functional motor activities from the positional base	Skilled action
Ability to move between different positions	Gross functional movement
Ease with which more complex functional movements (e.g. those involving upper limb or head movement during ambulation) can be attempted or achieved	Automatic execution and adaptation of sophisticated functional movement

findings, it is useful to prefix what was found on the day of assessment with any relevant or contextual information. This may be to refer the reader to other sections of the report, for example when performance is thought to have been influenced by low mood, or when the physical assessment, and therefore the validity of the picture being described, has been limited by behavioural factors. Other global influencing factors such as the impact of pain or dizziness, or limitations caused by such things as fractured limbs or the wearing of appliances, should also be recorded.

Performance in sitting

Description of functional performance can be helped by considering in detail a checklist of questions derived from knowledge of biomechanics, postural control and skilled motor performance. Suggestions for further reading in this regard are given at the end of this chapter. The following are examples of deductive questions that may be used to establish any variance from normal ability in sitting.

Was the individual able to achieve a balanced sitting position?

Was support or assistance required in any way? Was the assistance provided by the environment, an external aid or a compensatory motor behaviour? How would you describe their optimum performance; what was the best sitting position observed? Did they achieve alignment of all body segments? Was there observable asymmetry or malalignment and, if so, where and in what plane? Was there any observable movement disorder at rest, or on movement? Was there any apparent soft tissue adaptation; what was its nature? Could this be influenced within the assessment? Was the malalignment caused by the soft tissue adaptation or was the malalignment a factor in the production of the soft tissue abnormalities? What other *causal* factors were identified during observation, examination or palpation?

Was the individual able to maintain their optimum position over time?

If sitting was achieved with apparently minimal effort, was it maintained to the same standard over time? Was the person being assessed aware of positional drift or was it necessary to alert them via external prompting? How was reorientation attempted; was it successful? Did the performance of head or limb movement have an effect on equilibrium? What about movements in the surrounding environment observed within their visual field; was their balance compromised by activity external to themselves? Was there evidence of excessive fixation to maintain safety?

Could they alter their centre of pressure on command or appropriate to task?

Was there appropriate reciprocal adjustment during weight displacement to maintain safety and to allow movement appropriate to the set task?

What was the level and quality of head and limb movement?

What about the speed, coordination and precision of the movements; were movements appropriately graded? How did isolated joint movement compare with multijoint activity? Could both arms be used in cooperation with each other? Was there any difference in movements performed close to the body and those performed at stretch? Was there any difference between free movements, those that were task directed or those requiring anticipatory postural response? Was there any observable movement disorder at rest or on movement? How was vision used during movement; were eye movements full and coordinated?

Was the level of performance influenced by the provision of support or external assistance?

Was it enhanced or hampered; in what way? Could performance be enhanced by any other intervention?

Movement into standing

In the same way, questions may be derived from knowledge of normal strategies used to rise into standing from a variety of sitting positions.

Was there adequate preparation before standing?

Did the person move towards symmetrical weight distribution; were the heels placed adequately posterior to the knees with full contact between feet and supporting surface? Was preparation attempted but not adequately achieved? Was a causal factor identified (soft tissue restriction, inadequate or excessive muscle activity, difficulty identifying the midline)?

Was horizontal (forward) weight transference initiated and continued to effect thigh-off?

Did the person exert and maintain sufficient pressure through both heels to achieve adequate forward propulsion? Did the knees move forward and down over the feet, the upper trunk forward and down? How did activity compare bilaterally; was progression achieved maintaining equilibrium, was pre-existing asymmetry accentuated or corrected? Were compensatory motor behaviours used to compensate for deficits or were premature saving reactions or manoeuvres to recover equilibrium in evidence? Did any other factor interfere with the free execution of the movement?

Was a smooth transition to the extension phase of standing up achieved?

Was there appropriate braking of the forward momentum? Was there adequate extension of the upper trunk, knee, hip and ankle?

How did the arms behave during standing from sitting?

Were they free to move forward? Did they remain relaxed? Were they used to aid propulsion?

Performance in standing

The maintenance of equilibrium in standing is a prerequisite for mobile function. Standing of itself has little functional value, but how an individual maintains a relatively static standing position and the success with which background control is adapted in response to changes in demand for postural orientation can provide a great deal of insight into the probability of achieving a multitude of functional tasks without directly assessing all such tasks.

A logical series of questions, following a similar thought process to that presented for sitting, can be used to structure the observation of symmetry, alignment, the access to limb movement, the quality of the movement available, the level of automatic postural adjustment and other functionally important components of skilled motor performance such as hand–eye coordination.

It may also be pertinent to observe and comment upon the conditions required to maintain standing in order to define the individual's maximal ability. For example, an individual's equilibrium may become vulnerable when vision is unavailable, or if required to perform a physical or cognitive task, or when required to respond at speed or without warning.

Gait and whole-body coordination

The final core heading in terms of basic motor performance relates to the ability to coordinate whole-body movement for mobility and higher level function. Much of the postural background will have already been described in sitting and standing, as will gross access to single limb movement. The description of gait should outline how the various abilities and deficits are integrated and how the demands of coordinating what should be a largely automatic motor skill are met.

Communication of findings to others will be enhanced if observations are placed in the context of normal reciprocal gait (see Further reading), allowing the globally familiar gait cycle to provide a basic structure. In addition to the discussion of the basic components of the gait cycle such as swing and stance phase, stride length, heel strike and toe-off, consideration should also be given to aspects of normal gait adaptability such as the automatic adjustment of stride length during directional change, the expectation of decreased double support time concomitant with increased walking velocity (and vice versa), and the increased upper body lag relative to the ipsilateral hip and pelvis associated with increasing walking velocity.

The assessment process that underpins such a description needs to explore the ability to deal with a wide set of ambulatory demands, at least to the level where confident inference can be made. The majority of people who sustain a TBI and present for rehabilitation are young and they require the ability to walk at various speeds in a variety of weather conditions and over a variety of terrains to return to a normally varied lifestyle. They also have to be able to *do* and to *think* while they walk. All these normal parameters need to be considered before establishing their true mobility level.

It is likely that in synthesizing the information gathered in the process of the assessment, certain movement characteristics emerge as common within a variety of functional movements; such characteristics or the compensatory strategies used to overcome them will usually be evident in the gait pattern. For example, there may a general reduction or absence of the rotational components of movement, or a consistent malalignment of the upper trunk segment over the pelvis, or even consistently poorly regulated movements either with regard to timing or to the exertion of force. Thus, if the failure of rotation is a limiting factor in the speed of gait that can be achieved, or if the individual can walk *only* at speed owing to difficulty in achieving stability around the hip and pelvis, this link should be explained along with the description of the gait.

Describing the abilities of the minimally active individual

Within this approach to reporting motor performance, a degree of antigravity function is identified as the defining factor in describing independent functional movement; this is given emphasis in beginning the description of motor performance in the context of the ability to sit up and free the upper limbs or head for functional movement. This delineation is deliberate as it forces the therapist and the reader to put the motor function available in the context of the level of independence open to the individual being assessed in terms of freedom from both human and environmental support.

However, having acknowledged what true independent motor performance is, it is essential, when assessing an individual whose abilities in some way fall short of the defined criteria, to detail the *components of activity* that are present. In addition, and to be consistent in maintaining a functional contextual bias, it is useful for the significance and the potential functional application of even minimal abilities to be given emphasis.

There are a number of objectives to be achieved by identifying even a single volition movement, describing the optimal circumstances in which it can be consistently performed or elicited, and suggesting how the movement may be used in a functional context. In individuals who are minimally responsive, the presence of such a reliable response can help to establish that they are able to relate in some way to the external environment, and in some cases can form the basis of a system of communication. For others who have access to more movement, for example of a single limb, but who nevertheless are limited by a lack of background control to use the movement in a constructive way, it is essential to identify and describe the position(s) and extent of postural support required to turn this into assisted function.

This focus on the detail of possible, albeit limited, function is somewhat in contrast to a more conventional description of function in lying, which so often hinges around whether or not the person being assessed can roll from side to side. Bed mobility and preparation to come into the sitting position are of undoubted functional importance, but if on assessment this level of motor performance is found to be beyond the individual it is not sufficient simply to report these negative findings without describing what that individual can do, as well as offering an explanation of what prevents them from doing more. In the same way, while recognizing that they may require maximum assistance to be placed in sitting, and sophisticated methods of maintaining the position, even such things as the ability to follow movement or other stimuli with their eyes should be recorded as a positive finding.

Physiotherapists do routinely observe this level of detail and they will often be responsible for the organization and maintenance of a functionally optimal sitting position. However, these types of rich data are rarely included in assessment reports, and the lack of documentation of progression through the subcomponents of functional movement at all levels of motor ability limits recognition of small but significant aspects of progress by therapists themselves and by others who audit the results of our endeavours.

Further considerations in relation to those performing at a high level

Physiotherapists are in the main unlikely to be called upon to assess those following TBI who are walking without aid and who have no obvious gross limb dysfunction. However, when, by virtue of the type of service that is being offered, an opinion is sought as to whether there is a physical basis for apparent underperformance or avoidance of physical activity, the freely ambulant patient can present one of the biggest challenges to a therapist's movement analysis and interpretative skills.

Of particular difficulty in setting comparative norms for this subsection of the TBI population is the apparently wide range of biomechanical profiles within the normal population. It is important, therefore, to ensure that assessment of the high-level performer is set in the context of their preinjury activity levels, motor habits, and work and leisure pursuits.

Following the direct physical assessment, borderline cases (when performance falls within what might be the low to middle range for age-related subjects) can often be clarified by discussion with relatives or friends, who will confirm the difference in the movement pattern or otherwise. Increasingly, family videos can be accessed for comparison. Also, in terms of interpretation, an average performance would not be consistent with normality when the preinjury history highlights involvement in regular and varied sporting activities or a work history that clearly demanded specific physical skills.

The issue may be, as often when assessing people following TBI, how much emphasis should be given to an individual's own report. Clinical experience is that, even in relatively minor injuries and in the presence of relatively minor cognitive dysfunction, self-assessment with regard to physical function is rarely realistic before specific attempts to return to previous levels of physical activity have been made. Those who have sustained the injury and their family and friends, particularly when the external evidence of the injury is limited, tend to expect to progress towards everything in time and do not anticipate difficulties in advance. Therefore, if the report is of no physical problems, it should be established whether this is based on experience or simply represents the fact that nothing has yet posed a difficulty in physical terms.

When gross global or local neurological deficits are not an issue, both the nervous system and the cardiovascular system need to be stressed before being given a clean bill of health. Functional tests of speed of response, whole-body coordination and balance should be combined with assessment of flexibility, exercise tolerance and other basic fitness indicators. In addition, subjective reports of inordinate levels of fatigue should be regarded as a potential indicator of a high-level movement inefficiency or difficulty with sensorimotor processing, and not simply assumed as being purely cognitively based.

There is increasing evidence of a close interrelationship between physical and cognitive performance, including the positive impact of physical exercise on cognitive performance. While experimental work in this area is still ongoing, the implication of such a direct link, combined with the issues discussed in terms of the integration of sensory information in the previous section, seem to argue strongly for increased involvement of the physiotherapy profession in the rehabilitation of people with minor TBI.

LIFE SKILLS

Finally, having set the context in terms of psychological well-being, deficits and abilities, a description of the person's *actual* functional level can be given including, where appropriate, reasons for any limitations or compensatory behaviours. In this way, the psychological, cognitive and physical contributions to suboptimal function are brought together.

Comments are divided into three main areas, which, as before, has the effect of both differentiating levels of ability and highlighting areas that are yet to be tested. For example, the assessment of someone who remains fully hospitalized cannot include definitive comment on *actual* ability to manage home finances or describe progress with community mobility. This delineation between predicted ability based on standardized tests and actual ability when in a real-life setting recognizes the limitations of standardized tests and stresses the multifactorial nature of successful life function.

PERSONAL CARE

Depending on the assessment venue, the level of independence in all aspects of personal care can be assessed by observation and/or the report of the individual and those immediately involved in a caring role. As an inpatient, information may be gathered from nursing assistants, other healthcare workers or family members who are contributing to care, while for those based at home discussions with partners or parents are often enlightening.

A semistructured interview will ensure that all cognitive and physical aspects are considered so as not to underestimate the level of assistance being given, for example in choosing or matching clothes, in prompting to bathe or shower, or via established habits of avoiding clothes with difficult fastenings.

HOME MANAGEMENT

It is important to establish the *actual* contribution to household management that the individual being assessed is making and whether this is in any way different from before the injury. Stereotypical division of roles cannot be assumed and even where, for example, someone would not regularly be the person who cooked the family meal, it is important to know whether this previously intact skill has been put to the test.

The relative importance of a variety of home management skills for each individual should be understood from the information gathered and described in the Lifestyle section. It may be that within the person's present home circumstances, and those anticipated for the immediate future, they will have no need to budget, plan meals or keep the laundry up to date. However, the lack of need to test or develop these basic skills for survival should not be confused with a presumption that the skills will automatically be there should such a need develop in the future. The true position should therefore be made clear in the wording of this section of the report.

COMMUNITY SKILLS

This last section of the main report should outline the scope of community activity being undertaken and the level of independence in relation to these activities. The influence of previously described difficulties or limitations should be described, including any cumulative effects. It is also useful to highlight any difference in ability levels for routine and new activities and, where known, to include details of the level of assistance given to establish current ability levels and any background support involved in maintaining the current level of function.

The processes by which the findings of this type of global assessment can be summarized and by which recommendations, including priority goals for intervention, can be developed will be considered in the next chapter.

REFERENCES

Ashburn A, members of the Motor Club 1982 A physical assessment of stroke patients. Physiotherapy 68:109–113

Berman J M, Fredrickson J M 1978 Vertigo after head injury: a five year follow-up. Journal of Otolaryngology 7:237–245

Brazzelli M, Della Sala S 1997 Physiotherapy and neuropsychology: an interaction that could ease the remedy of brain disease. Physiotherapy Theory and Practice 13:243–246

Bronstein A 1995 Visual vertigo syndrome: clinical and posturography findings. Journal of Neurology, Neurosurgery and Psychiatry 59(5):472–476

Carey L M, Oke L, Matyas T A 1996 Impaired limb position sense after stroke: a quantitative test for clinical use. Archives of Physical Medicine and Rehabilitation 77: 1271–1278

Carey L M, Oke L, Matyas T A 1997 Impaired touch discrimination after stroke: a quantitative test. Journal of Neurologic Rehabilitation 11:219–232

Carpenter R H S 1996 The control of posture. In: Neurophysiology, 3rd edn. Arnold, London, ch 11, p 214

Clarke F, Horch K W, Bach S, Larson G 1979 Contributions of cutaneous and joint receptors to static position sense in man. Journal of Neurophysiology 42(3):877–888

Clarke F, Burgess R, Chapin J, Lipscomb W 1985 Role of intramuscular receptors and the awareness of limb position. Journal of Neurophysiology 6):1529–1540

Curthoys I, Baloh R 1995 Vestibular compensation: a review of the oculomotor, neural and clinical consequences of unilateral vestibular loss. Journal of Vestibular Research 5:67–107 de Jong P T V M, de Jong J M B, Cohen B, Jongkees L B W 1976 Ataxia and nystagmus induced by injection of local anesthetics in the neck. Annals of Neurology 1:240–246

Gandevia S, McCloskey D, Burke D 1992 Kinesthetic signals and muscle contraction. Trends in Neuroscience 15(2):62–65

Herdman S J 1994 Vestibular rehabilitation, 1st edn. FA Davis, Philadelphia, PA

Karlberg M 1995 The neck and human balance: a clinical and experimental approach to 'cervical vertigo'. University Hospital of Lund, Lund

Lincoln N, Leadbitter D 1979 Assessment of motor function in stroke patient. Physiotherapy 65:48–51

Lincoln N, Crow J, Jackson J et al 1991 The unreliability of sensory assessments. Clinical Rehabilitation 5:273–282

Mawson S J 1993 Measuring physiotherapy outcome in stroke rehabilitation. Physiotherapy 79:762–765

Nashner L 1993 Computerised dynamic posturography. In: Jacobson G, Newman C, Kartush J (eds) Handbook of balance function testing. Mosby, St Louis, MI, p 280

Shepard N T, Telian S A 1996 Practical management of the balance disorder patient, 1st edn. Singular Publishing, San Diego, CA

Shumway-Cook A 1994 Vestibular rehabilitation in traumatic brain injury. In: Herdman S (ed) Vestibular rehabilitation, 1st edn. FA Davis, Philadelphia, PA, p 347

Shumway-Cook A, Horak F 1986 Assessing the influence of sensory interaction on balance. Physical Therapy 66:1881–1885

Sim J, Waterfield J 1997 Validity, reliability and responsiveness in the assessment of pain. Physiotherapy Theory and Practice 13:23–37

Sluka K A, Rees H 1997 The neuronal response to pain. Physiotherapy Theory and Practice 13:3–22

Van Deusen J, Foss J J 1997 Sensory deficits. In: Van Deusen J, Brunt D (eds) Assessment in occupational therapy and physical therapy, 1st edn. WB Saunders, Philadelphia, PA, p 296

Voorhees R 1989 The role of dynamic posturography in neurotological diagnosis. Laryngoscope 99:940–957

Voorhees R 1990 Dynamic posturography findings in central nervous system disorders. Laryngoscope 100:995–1001

Wilkins A 1995 Visual stress, 1st edn. Oxford Scientific Publications, Oxford

Winward C, Wade D, Halligan P 1998 Somatosensory performance: assessment after stroke. Poster presentation to a conference on Human motor performance: the interaction between science and therapy, University of East London, London, 21–23 July 1998

Zee D 1994 Vestibular adaptation. In: Herdman S J (ed) Vestibular rehabilitation, 1st edn. FA Davis, Philadelphia, PA, p 68

FURTHER READING

Abernethy B, Kippers V, Mackinnon L T, Neal R J, Hanrahan S 1996 The biophysical foundations of human movement. Human Kinetics, Champaign, IL

Latash M L 1998 Neurophysiological basis of movement. Human Kinetics, Champaign, IL

Magill R A 1993 Motor learning: concepts and applications, 4th edn. Brown & Benchmark, Madison, WI

Roberts T D M 1995 Understanding balance – the mechanisms of posture and locomotion. Chapman & Hall, London

Rosenbaum D A 1991 Human motor control. Academic Press, San Diego, CA

Rothwell J 1994 Control of human voluntary movement, 2nd edn. Chapman & Hall, London

Whittle M 1991 Gait analysis: an introduction. Butterworth–Heinemann, London

Winter D A 1990 Biomechanics and motor control of human movement, 2nd edn. John Wiley, New York

7

Defining goals for intervention

Key Points

- The collation and cross-referencing of assessment findings is an integral part of the assessment process, and within an interdisciplinary model of working this should take place in advance of the identification of intervention goals
- Goal setting involves consideration of the assessment findings in the context of knowledge of the natural history of TBI, locally available resources and the remit of the service
- The combined process of discussing assessment findings and defining goals for intervention is best achieved by following a predetermined structure based on clearly defined objectives
- Although programme goals are formulated within the team, and with thorough assessment should reflect the goals of the injured individual, these targets and the proposed means of achieving them need to be agreed directly with the client, recorded and reviewed

COMPLETING THE PRIMARY ASSESSMENT PROCESS

Within an interdisciplinary approach, the process of goal setting is based around pooling knowledge of the natural history of traumatic brain injury (TBI), the locally available resources and the remit of the service, together with the findings of the assessment process. As has been described in some detail, the assessment process should comprise direct and indirect methods of information gathering from many sources and with regard to a wide range of factors.

This process generates different levels of data. Some of the data are factual and have a clear meaning independent of other information. Some, as in the case of information gathered by a number of observers via a structured checklist, are designed to be considered together. Other information, exemplified by the assessment of cognition, needs to be compared and contrasted with other findings to help establish accurate understanding of the type of deficit and its severity, and to anticipate the functional implications for the individual being assessed.

This process of confirming assessment findings can be usefully linked with the discussion of appropriate intervention and/or management goals so that resultant recommendations are consistent with the pathology, the stage of recovery, the resources available and the strengths, limitations and aspirations of the person being assessed.

INFORMATION SHARING AND DISCUSSION

The interdisciplinary discussions and practice development that produced the initial assessment report template upon which the preceding chapters are closely modelled also identified the need for informal and formal communication systems to use the time available for the initial assessment efficiently, and to share and cross-reference the gathered information in a concise way. Thus, the content of the assessment pro forma used to standardize the gathering of information before and during the assessment process was generated and agreed by all team members.

To some extent, the fact that the service within which this all developed was community based and covered a wide geographical area forced the development of a concise, time-limited initial assessment while still attempting to cover enough ground to develop a global picture of the individual being assessed. In the same way, a high level of service demand did not allow time for open-ended discussion, necessitating the development of a highly structured, goal-oriented assessment discussion meeting.

There is a body of opinion which says that interdisciplinary working is a luxury that subacute inpatient rehabilitation units with a high turnover of patients cannot afford. This argument is based mainly around time and organizational factors, and particularly the beliefs that discussion is time consuming and that it is often difficult to get all team members in the same place at the same time.

It should be recognized that all services have particular time and organizational pressures and a variety of other limiting factors within which they have to operate. The art in making interdisciplinary working fit within the constraints of any service is to limit the extent of information gathering, discussion and goal setting to that which is relevant to the expected period of contact and the stage of recovery of the individual (see Ch. 4). In this way the principles of interdisciplinary global assessment can be retained without the process becoming unwieldy and bureaucratic.

However, whatever the extent of the assessment process, the nature of interdisciplinary working demands that there is discussion of findings across the team in *advance* of setting specific goals, so that priorities and a common approach can be agreed. This is in contrast to multidisciplinary working when individual practitioners share with colleagues their previously formulated goals and keep one another informed of progress on a regular basis.

INTERDISCIPLINARY ASSESSMENT CASE DISCUSSION

The interdisciplinary assessment case discussion has specific objectives but it also brings additional benefits. The primary objectives within the assessment structure already described are to:

- Confirm that all relevant records have been accessed and that a clear medical and progress history has been obtained and is understood by all team members
- Review (briefly) the findings in relation to the core skills assessment, highlighting ability level and areas of concern
- Discuss those issues reliant on multiple informants and those requiring clarification via cross-referencing or exploratory discussion
- Review or discuss the psychosocial findings and, in particular, establish the individual's level of awareness (insight)
- Identify possible areas for intervention with reference to
  - the concerns and/or goals described by the individual and, when appropriate, the carers
  - the viewpoint of the professionals
- Prioritize intervention foci, taking into account such things as
  - core skills and factors that underpin many functions
  - motivating factors
  - appropriate programme intensity
  - the need for further assessment
  - projected medium- and long-term goals
  - projected period of contact
  - potential barriers to successful intervention
- Identify a key worker (primary therapist, case coordinator) and a second named person to offer backup to the key worker.

In addition to achieving the primary objectives, the nature and content of the discussion also makes the meeting an educational forum, sharing disciplinary knowledge, promoting understanding of alternative methods of working, offering opportunities to question and, sometimes, highlighting particular topic areas that can be followed up at other times. This all contributes to staff and team development.

Becoming skilled and efficient within this process as an individual and as a team requires an appropriate structure and a fair degree of application. In terms of structure, having one person chair the meeting, ensuring coverage of the predetermined agenda and equity of time for discussion of all the necessary topics is key to efficiency. As well as good time management skills, the person chairing needs to understand the global assessment process and be able to facilitate clarity of discussion.

A separate person (not directly involved in the assessment) to make summary written notes is equally important to ensure that the salient points of the discussion are recorded for future reference and that agreed action is clearly documented.

PRIORITIZING ISSUES WITHIN THE TEAM

When there is good team working within a service that has a clear remit or is based around a common vision, the range of potential management or intervention goals will emerge in the course of discussion. Priority issues can then be agreed with reference to the broad-brush list of influential factors already given.

However, the concept of not *automatically* intervening following an assessment that reveals physical dysfunction is, I believe, alien to many physiotherapists. In addition, the nature of the sensorimotor deficits encountered after TBI often argues strongly for intervention, at the very least to prevent secondary physical developments that would have a negative impact on future functional ability. In practice, the occasions when other interventions take complete priority over physical issues are relatively rare but equally, in the face of other deficits that have great import in terms of functional independence, physiotherapists do have to consider, along with other team members, the relative balance of the planned interventions.

This process, and the thinking that accompanies it, can open up many possibilities to combine treatment strategies, follow complementary programmes and reinforce various types of information being given to the person who is the focus of the rehabilitation programme and to all those who perform supporting roles. All of these facets, common recognizable strategies, reinforcement and repetition are positive factors for learning in the normal and pathological state. In addition, where goals of intervention can be related directly or indirectly to real-life functional tasks or outcomes recognized as important by the injured person, positive motivational factors are added, along with the clear possibility of achieving regular practice in everyday life.

The mechanics of this process of defining and prioritizing goals are illustrated via Case examples 7.1–7.3 which follow. The main events common to negotiating and agreeing a programme of intervention are then reviewed.

Case example 7.1   Barbara

Brief background and status

Twenty-year-old female, injured in road traffic accident. Diffuse closed head injury, lowest Glasgow Coma Score (GCS) 3, in coma for 5 months. Now 10 months postinjury. No previous medical history.

Lifestyle

Preinjury: In nurse training, living away from home. Loved music, clothes and socializing. Keen swimmer.
Now: Soon to be discharged to live with parents; no social life except for occasional clothes-shopping trips. Sister visits.

Psychosocial issues

Behavioural problems recorded in clinical notes; parents deny any problems in this area. Language difficulties limit formal assessment, flattened affect observed, smiled at male staff member, one (very) aggressive outburst during assessment, objected to being assisted to transfer on to toilet even though unable to do this on her own.

Core skills

Mainly low arousal, poor attention. Fatigue evident, three major rest periods during the full day of assessment.
Occasional single word utterance, no apparent recognition of the written word, ?visual/perceptual problems. Responds to her name and appears to take cues from gesture and context. Loud vocalization and strong shaking of left hand to express annoyance/anger; not graded.
Unable to sit without support, high tone and limited range throughout right side and tactile defensive.
Autobiographical recall (at least partial) evident by response to family pictures and possessive handling of a nurse's hat acquired from a nurse on the hospital ward. Family believe that she recalls happenings from day to day, hospital staff are less sure.

Integrative skills

No opportunity to observe; major problems with core skills.

Functional level

Tries to assist with personal care; wears loose, adapted clothing. Can use spoon and cup in left hand. Needs one to transfer, two when tired.

Key factors in planning initial intervention

Parental home 40-min car journey from rehabilitation centre. Able to concentrate for only 15 min at a time. Parents keen to have her home and want rehab from specialist unit.

Additional information required

Visual testing. Possibility of delaying home discharge.

Case example 7.1   *Cont'd*

Recommended initial programme

Physical programme to desensitize right side and achieve unsupported sitting. Graded cognitive stimulation programme. Planned time-limited sessions, mornings only, alternate days, alternate physical/cognitive first thing.

Further envisaged programme

Review response to programme in 3 months. If positive, further 18 months to 2 years of involvement anticipated. Unlikely to progress to independent living, very unlikely to return to nursing.

Discussion of Case example 7.1

These are the immediate external influencing factors in the decision-making process facing the team in Barbara's case. Discharge from the inpatient facility has been promised and the assessing service has been described to Barbara's parents as the best place for outpatient rehabilitation. Therefore, although extended inpatient rehabilitation or an outpatient service requiring less travel would better suit her stamina and concentration level, neither of these recommendations is acceptable to Barbara's parents.

There is an unspoken impression gained from Barbara's parents that they believe she would be doing better with higher quality intervention. There is also a conflict of opinion regarding the appropriateness of some of Barbara's behaviours, with her parents reporting no personal experience of any inappropriate behaviour, in contrast to a number of events recorded in the clinical records.

The assessing team considers that Barbara's parents cannot yet comprehend the severity of her injury and probably have unrealistic expectations of the outcome from the rehabilitation programme. A common approach to information giving is therefore adopted to give consistent clear messages that the injury severity means that Barbara's life will be very different from that planned before, but that the team want to work together with Barbara and her family to make her new life as positive and independent as possible.

An honest but caring relationship with Barbara's parents is also seen as the key to tackling the difficult issue of inappropriate behaviours, which is anticipated as a potentially divisive issue between the professionals and the parents, but where consistency of approach will be key in managing any emerging behaviours. Therefore, while only limited progress is anticipated directly with Barbara over the initial period of attendance while her stamina and concentration are developed, this period is seen as being key in developing mutual trust for what will be a long and hard period of subsequent rehabilitation.

To monitor progress clearly, to pace demands and to limit fatigue-related negative behaviours, it is decided to structure working sessions. Initially, each 40-min session is split into 15 min of work, 10 min of rest and 15 min of work.

Sessions to work on Barbara's motor performance and self-care skills are placed first on alternate days of attendance to allow Barbara to be fresh for each treatment focus on an equal basis. This is because second sessions (even after a rest period) will achieve less than would be achieved in a first session, and it is hoped to prevent an unequal emphasis on one intervention and avoid alienation caused by fatigue.

Structured observation of communicative behaviours is planned to take place within a variety of sessions. Joint therapeutic sessions are also included regularly in the timetable.

As well as the demands of travel being taken into account in limiting attendance, the transition to home life is also recognized as significant. Barbara and her family need to spend some time together (in the absence of professionals) to allow the development of a more realistic assessment of her functional level. As stamina improves, attendance at therapy can increase, giving additional respite for the family.

The intervention goals are therefore:

1. To structure intervention at an optimal level so that constructive stimulus is achieved without provoking fatigue related behavioural difficulties
2. To develop a relationship of mutual trust and respect with Barbara and her parents as a base for future negotiations and decision making, and to promote consistency of approach
3. To monitor and record negative behaviours, their provoking factors and their resolution
4. To achieve right-side lying without distress, initial time target of 15 min
5. To achieve sitting, symmetrical at pelvic level, therapist sitting on right, Barbara tolerating handling of right arm and hand
6. To achieve sustained visual attention (initial time target of 15 min) and visual tracking from left to right
7. To investigate basic visual perceptual skills, colour, shape, etc.
8. To promote bilateral function in line with progress on 4, 5, 6 and 7
9. To monitor and evaluate functional communication in a variety of real-life settings
10. To develop a further action plan based on response to therapy over a 2–3-month period.

Case example 7.2   Bryan

Brief background and status

Forty-five-year-old man, injured in a road traffic accident. Lowest GCS recorded as 12; not initially scanned or detained in hospital. Fractured left clavicle, frontotemporal facial lacerations. Now 12 months postinjury. General practitioner (GP) had tried to get Bryan to go back to work 1 month after injury. No intervening contact with health services. Previous history of surgery for eye squint.

Lifestyle

Preinjury: Government employee and part-time soldier. Independent and very active. Steady partner in a different city.
Now: Living with partner, at home most of the time, does not go out alone.

Psychosocial issues

Partner reports him as irritable and verbally aggressive but also withdrawn for long periods of time. Anxious in public, sometimes verbally inappropriate, apparently unaware of the impact of his behaviour on others. High scores on tests of anxiety and depression. Guilty about not returning to work.

Core skills

Good focused attention with suggestion of difficulty disengaging. Fatigue apparent in performance on cognitive testing. Good vocabulary and understanding of verbal language but reports major negative change in reading ability. Recall of new information extremely poor on testing, verbal and visual, occasionally helped by prompts. Self-reported difficulty with names and faces. High-level left-sided weakness, painful and restricted left shoulder and neck. Poor balance, dizziness, headaches.

Integrative skills

Performed well on an assessed (previously habitual) kitchen task but unable to evaluate his own performance and felt he did not do well. Obviously fatigued after task. Returned home and slept for rest of afternoon (had to be wakened). Difficulty with decision-making/choices on formal testing. Unable to handle monetary transactions.

Functional level

Slow but mostly independent in self-care. Unable to match clothes (previously snappy dresser). Had made occasional successful journey by bus in city where he grew up but had also got lost on more than one occasion. No longer goes out on his own.

Key factors in planning initial intervention

Education to promote understanding of reasons why he has genuinely not been able to return to work. Establish clearer picture of frequency and functional impact of subjective complaints. Establish knowledge of pattern of activities and relationship with subjective complaints.

Additional information required

Medical evaluation of ?absence attacks. Ophthalmological opinion on eyes.

Recommended initial programme

Physical programme (face validity with Bryan). Establish strategies for recording activities and then memory support. Education about TBI and effects to be interwoven.

Case example 7.2   *Cont'd*

Further envisaged programme

Review programme after 6 weeks, ?impact of decreased anxiety on cognitive performance. Likely involvement/prognosis difficult to predict; assessment performance poorer than expected from available history.

Discussion of Case example 7.2

Bryan's assessment raised as many questions as it answered. The medical records relating to the initial injury were minimal and focused on the left shoulder injury. The facial lacerations were recorded but, other than the paramedic's record of GCS 12, no further reference was made to a TBI.

A neurological opinion at 6 weeks postinjury estimated post-traumatic amnesia at less than 10 hours and suggested that post-traumatic stress disorder was the main factor in Bryan not having returned to work. The rehabilitation team's assessment suggested significant cerebral damage (based on cognitive and physical findings) and a more substantial period of post-traumatic amnesia, possibly up to the time Bryan was seen by the neurologist.

Although it was seen as important to establish in detail the level of Bryan's cognitive performance, especially because of the apparent discrepancy, the initial intervention was judged to be best built around a physical programme because it was thought that he would respond to an immediately recognizable, concrete objective that related to his preinjury self-image. This was a man who had run a half-marathon in the weeks before his injury and who had just passed his annual medical to remain an active part-time soldier.

On assessment Bryan could not maintain a 'static' standing position, even with eyes open, or sit without upper limb support. His sleep was disturbed every night by severe vertiginous episodes and he suffered from recurrent headaches. Even with these tangible difficulties and the additional cognitive problems that he reported, Bryan was still preoccupied by wanting to be back at work and by having been told by his GP that he should be back at work. At the same time he would express that he knew he could not cope with the physical or mental demands of his job and he was aggrieved by his GP's apparent lack of understanding.

Further detailed exploration of the physical signs and subjective complaints, along with their response to treatment, would inform the longer-term physical programme and provide a basis for Bryan's understanding of the link between his difficulties and the fact that he was not yet at work. Although he had performed consistently poorly on several formal tests of memory and learning, he was only really complaining of difficulty remembering people's names.

Bryan's partner's report suggested that she thought he was selective in his memory loss and there were obvious tensions in her interpretation of his behaviour in general. Neither she nor Bryan had had any specific education or support regarding the effects of TBI, and the limited professional contact that they did have was suggestive of Bryan making more of the situation than was reasonable. The particular insistence by the GP that Bryan should be back at work caused him eventually to change his doctor, which had resulted in the referral for assessment.

It was decided that it would be useful to obtain a clear picture of activity levels at home and that this could be linked to recording the frequency and association of headache and dizziness, which was also required for the physical programme. The plan was to use the process of gathering the information and the resultant detail as a focus for the development of a cognitive programme, developing functional goals around which to pin further assessment and intervention.

Bryan's partner was offered direct support from a specialist TBI social worker, to allow bilateral development of greater understanding of her experience and of the functional effects of TBI deficits to facilitate collaborative working later in the rehabilitation programme. Therefore, the goals for intervention were to:

- Use the physical programme as a vehicle to
  - improve physical performance (symmetrical, aligned sitting without upper limb support and with a freely moving head; steady standing without upper limb support)
  - decrease negative symptoms (dizziness in supine and side lying, headache)
  - gain a clear picture of the factors provoking negative symptoms and therefore the management principles to work towards their resolution
  - investigate eye movement and the functional use of visual feedback
  - provide a functional (motivating) reason to record home-based activity to help inform the development of a wider rehabilitation programme
  - validate the functional impact of Bryan's injury and promote a more equitable self-assessment of his present non-working status
- Use the development and structure of a recording system to
  - provide information detail and feedback on the results of physical treatments
  - highlight to Bryan and his partner the functional impact of his cognitive problems
  - develop a home-based exercise habit
  - identify functional goals around which to develop the wider rehabilitation programme
  - reduce working memory demands and influence anxiety levels

Case example 7.3   Hamid

Brief background and status

Eighteen-year-old male, injured in road traffic accident. Lowest GCS 5, multiple facial fractures, major reconstructive surgery. Inpatient for 6 weeks. Now 4 months' postinjury. History of back injury at age 12 years.

Lifestyle

Preinjury: Living with older brother; just started college. Keen basketball player. Now: Living with parents; another brother has learning difficulties. Spends much of the day in bed.

Psychosocial issues

Withdrawn. Minimal eye contact throughout assessment. No initiation of conversations (even at home). Parents think he is distressed by facial appearance (no obvious scars but nose flattened and eyes slightly malaligned).

Core skills

Great difficulties with attention (all aspects) and very slow processing on formal testing and in interactional behaviour. Difficulties with written and spoken language, but English not first language, ?how much an acquired problem. Absent sense of smell and taste. Severe headache and facially hypersensitive above temple level. Unable to fixate gaze, produces disorientation and dizziness. Poor truncal control, unable to sit without upper limb support although walking (wide base but not classically ataxic). Body segments malaligned in sagittal and frontal planes. Extremely poor memory across formal tests and structured tasks (did recall the kitchen incident detailed below, when prompted).

Integrative skills

Unable to attempt much of the formal testing. Set the pan alight during kitchen assessment and, although aware of the problem, managed only to take one step back and stare.

Functional level

Can physically dress if clothes clearly available. Washes only when prompted. No contribution to home management. Does not go out.

Key factors in planning initial Intervention

Reduction of headache, establish impact on performance. Provide reason to get out of bed and leave house. Lives a short walking distance from the rehabilitation centre.

Additional information required

Actual physical damage to eye muscles and bony sockets (how much of eye movement problem is centrally mediated?).

Recommended initial programme

Physical programme to test hypothesis that headache is referred from upper cervical dysfunction, decrease facial sensitivity; slowly increase treatment/length of activity sessions. Start work on attention when headache reduced.

Further envisaged programme

Review after 4 weeks. Medical review if headache no better; commence progressive cognitive and physical programme if positive response. Length of active rehabilitation programme dependent on evidence of ability to learn, period of contact anticipated as lengthy (2 years or more).

- Provide a forum for Bryan's partner to resolve some of her anger at being left to cope and, by education, develop a greater understanding of the functional impact of Bryan's deficits
- Develop a further action plan based on the response to intervention after 6 weeks.

Discussion of Case example 7.3

Hamid's performance across testing was very poor indeed, and the main question was whether any other factor was contributing to the overall poor performance. There were three main potential contributory factors. One was his complaint of headache, the second his apparent low mood and/or arousal, and the third was the potential impact of him being tested via a language that he had started to learn only as a young teenager. However, his family reported that he was equally slow to respond if addressed in his mother tongue and his performance on non-verbal tasks was equally poor, so language was thought not to be a primary factor. It was therefore decided to focus on the other two factors for a short initial period of intervention before mapping out a more detailed programme.

Since Hamid lived only a couple of minutes' walk away from the rehabilitation centre and there was a pedestrian crossing over the only busy road, the programme started with multiple short (20–30 min) attendances. At first he would be escorted by a family member and, when they judged him safe, he would walk to the centre on his own.

An additional consideration was that while he had his reportedly constant severe headache he would not be able to tolerate any useful period of intervention and, if the headache did not have a musculoskeletal provoking factor, further medical guidance would be paramount. Therefore, in this case, only the physical therapy programme commenced immediately after assessment, even though Hamid had major deficits in all core skill areas that would eventually need to be addressed.

The intervention goals were therefore identified as:

- To reduce the frequency and intensity of headache via manual therapy and exercise as appropriate
- To desensitize the skin of the upper face and head via therapist and self massage
- To increase intervention time from 20 min to up to 1 hour (if appropriate)
- To change the home-based inactive behaviour to at least one short daily outing

To develop a further action plan based on response to treatment over 4 weeks.

Overview of the three cases

In all three case studies the plan for initial intervention was developed by considering all the evidence including the practicalities of attendance and developmental work to facilitate future envisaged intervention. In two of the three cases, decisions regarding the approach and content of the programme were heavily influenced by the needs of the carers, as perceived by the professional staff.

While the service was not funded to work substantially with carers, a somewhat pragmatic stance was taken to try to ensure that involved carers (with client consent) would understand the rationale for the proposed programme and would, in effect, consent to the treatment approach and contribute appropriately towards its success. An active contribution in terms of direct therapy was not assumed and was in fact often discouraged, but carers were expected wherever possible to be consistent with the team approach and not to undermine the necessary work towards the targeted functional goals.

In some circumstances programme agreements were formalized via simple contracts, which could include family members as well as the client and staff involved.

COMMUNICATING RECOMMENDATIONS

Whether the planned programme is to be structured in the form of a contract or not, the assessment findings plus any questions raised by the assessment process and the specific recommendations being suggested for implementation need to be communicated to those who have taken part in the assessment. The initial part of this communication can take place at a meeting arranged for the purpose, to complete the assessment process but, given the complexity of many cases and the limitations on understanding caused by cognitive difficulties and emotional status, additional written and/or verbally presented material will usually be required.

THE FEEDBACK MEETING

As with the assessment case discussion, a formalized meeting to complete the initial assessment process has both specific objectives and provides additional opportunities. The main objectives of such a meeting are to:

- Summarize the main findings of the assessment
- If possible, explain the significance of the findings
- Gather additional information

- Raise issues requiring clarification and either resolve them or agree on the next step in trying to do so
- Receive feedback on the client and carers' experience of the assessment
- Allow further questions to be asked of the professional staff
- Put forward the team's recommended plan and set it in the context of projected goals and, where appropriate, anticipated outcome
- Introduce the concept of the key worker and identify the personnel involved
- Agree a plan of action

Agreeing primary goals

As has been illustrated in the case studies, the identification of the primary goals within the team is, in the end, a logical and practical process; with some practice and the support of other team members, it is relatively straightforward following a thorough assessment.

When the assessment is client based, the occasions when the suggested goals are not acceptable to the client and their families are rare, as lifestyle influences and personal aspirations will have been taken into account in the formulation of the goals. In the same way, if part of the problem is a discrepancy between perceived levels of deficit, for example a lack of awareness or an active denial of a problem, the team formulation will have included specific attention to these basic issues and they will be proposing an approach specifically to address this problem.

Rehabilitation goals are achievable only if everyone is working towards the same ideal, and one way or another the team's recommendations have to be 'sold' to the client and to any supporting personnel. This is done most easily if the goals are seen to be valid or are presented in the context of enabling a more complex valid goal.

Where the initial goals are far removed from the desired functional outcome, or the proposed intervention is abstract or difficult to understand, the offer of a time-limited review may give adequate reassurance that programmes are negotiable, and ultimately that the individual is not compelled to take part in any rehabilitation programme. However, if goals are renegotiated in some way or accepted on condition, it is important that what is eventually agreed is clearly recorded and that all concerned have access to a copy of that record.

Roles and responsibilities

As part of the immediate agreement and to ensure best practice throughout the period of contact, it is useful to define roles and responsibilities as they relate to specific programmes and to other processes that support the delivery and review of programmes. This may appear unnecessarily bureaucratic but it does help ensure that plans are actioned or, if found to be incomplete, the block or barrier is more easily identified. Also, within a busy service it aids staff recall; for clients with cognitive limitations it can be used as a reference point and, if and when there are points of dissatisfaction or misunderstanding, it can help introduce clarity into potentially emotional interactions.

The process of listing goals and assigning responsibilities makes the demands on clients, staff and others more tangible and so limits the occurrence of programmes that overestimate or underestimate the abilities of the client and should highlight commitments that are impossible for staff to deliver. In addition, the need for supplementary support from other sources should be more easily identified and requests for this support more straightforward to document. All of this introduces a degree of external control to potentially very fluid and unwieldy circumstances.

Review

When the structure and timing for review has been mapped out, every effort should be made to honour this agreement. If the plan cannot be implemented, this needs to be explained and a new plan agreed. It is important to be realistic in the expectations contained within each implementation and review plan, including the demands that such a plan places on team members. This realism also includes the need to acknowledge the limitations of the service on offer; in most services that means the need to include discussion of discharge planning from the very beginning of the process.

SUMMARY AND RECOMMENDATIONS

Finally, having discussed the assessment findings, agreed on the team priorities for intervention, and explained and agreed a plan of action with the individual under assessment, the broad findings and immediate plan can be recorded within the assessment report, completing the initial assessment process.

Designing interventions

SECTION CONTENTS

8

Applying neurophysiotherapeutic principles

Key Points

- The development of a sound theoretical base for neurophysiotherapeutic practice has been limited by inadequate knowledge of how exactly the neuromuscular system is controlled and regulated
- Historically, treatment techniques have been developed via clinical observation, trial and error, with clinically successful forms of intervention being passed on via an oral tradition
- There is a need for improved documentation and the collation of existing knowledge and scientific evidence to inform clinical practice and to assist movement towards a single theory of motor control and away from a multitude of treatment concepts
- Progress in these areas and in the development of an improved academic profile is dependent upon establishing effective communication between practitioners of different traditions, academics and researchers, and on each individual professional recognizing their responsibility to contribute to an open and constructive debate
- An open, inclusive framework for the analysis of evidence and the development of knowledge is proposed, and its application to TBI is demonstrated via clinical examples

HISTORICAL CONTEXT

Physiotherapy as a profession began its evolution little more than a century ago and it is only within the last 50 years that the move towards autonomous practice and specialization within the profession began. The origins of physiotherapy and its practice are strongly rooted in practical hands-on intervention with the use of adjunctive modalities such as electrotherapy and remedial exercise being incorporated into routine practice at an early stage in the development of the profession.

The majority of practice development across the various specialties within physiotherapy has, until relatively recent times, been achieved mainly through experiential learning, within the context of a sound knowledge of anatomy and physiology in health and disease. However, a basic problem for physiotherapists working in the field of neuropathology has been the global ignorance of how exactly the central nervous system (CNS), which we cannot see or touch, works and how it interrelates functionally with the peripheral musculoskeletal system, which we can observe and handle.

Within these limitations of knowledge, the means by which neurophysiotherapeutic treatments were developed were therefore primarily via physical exploration of the peripheral musculoskeletal system with the subsequent development of manual skills and/or exercise regimes, the effects of which had apparent face validity in the hospital or clinic. Commonly, when the particular developed approach to treatment was believed to have a positive effect, the associated techniques were then described and taught to other therapists.

Early neurophysiotherapeutic treatments were not, however, entirely without a theoretical base; for example, Rood (1954) and Kabat & Knott (1954) both cite the neurophysiological knowledge of the time as a basis for the treatment techniques described within their concepts. Other intuitive practitioners have attempted to explain their clinical success more in retrospect by citing experimental evidence; for example, Bobath (1978) cites the work of Magnus (1926), Sherrington (1913, 1947) and Beevor (1904), amongst others.

However, even though these limited connections between practice and evidence (and those described by the proponents of other treatment concepts) were described, clinical practice during the 1960s and 1970s to a large extent developed independently of scientific knowledge and mainly in response to observed clinical success. Moreover, during the same period, there was very little in the way of explanatory literature or documented evidence of outcome forthcoming from any of the schools of thought. Consequently, pre and post registration neurophysiotherapy education tended to emphasize the treatment technique, with only minimal reference to the evidential basis for treatment, and when attempts were made to link scientific knowledge and theory with current practice they appeared to be, to some extent, incompatible.

With hindsight, this is hardly surprising given that the then current theory of hard-wired hierarchical neural control of motor performance has been left behind by mounting evidence of distributed processing and neural plasticity. Certainly in the UK, and I suspect elsewhere, practice reflected this dissociated relationship between clinical activity and academic investigation, and the divide continued until the relatively recent past and continues to influence what is still an uneasy alliance.

A further difficulty that arose from the combination of minimal literature and the heavy reliance on cascaded teaching by individual practitioners was that what came to be practised under the various headings of say Bobath or proprioceptive neuromuscular facilitation (PNF) varied tremendously across practitioners and certainly across continents. In recent years attempts have been made to standardize postgraduate teaching and descriptive language, for example in relation to the Bobath concept, but while this and other treatment concepts continue to rely heavily on direct experiential teaching without adequate description in mainstream literature, significant developmental barriers remain. In particular there are problems in undertaking generalizable research (and therefore in establishing levels of efficacy) and there are no overt mechanisms for open discussion of emerging issues or for adding to the body of knowledge.

The link between scientific evidence, scholarly theories and clinical practice has been made more overtly and consistently by author-practitioners outside of the UK, most notably the Movement Science framework (Carr & Shepherd 1987, 1998) and the Systems Approach (Shumway-Cook & Woollacott 1995). For all of us, however, the combination of the spiralling cost of healthcare and a more knowledgeable and questioning public has focused our attention more than ever on what we do, why we do it and how effective it is.

CURRENT AND FUTURE PRACTICE

It is not the intention to provide a complete review of treatment philosophies and approaches within this chapter (for further historical and evaluative information see Partridge 1996, Plant 1998) or, indeed, to argue in favour of one particular established treatment approach. However, it should be self-evident from the content of this book so far that whatever physical treatment approach is employed within a rehabilitation or management programme for someone who has sustained a traumatic brain injury (TBI), it needs to be delivered within the context of the wider rehabilitation programme and with due attention to coexisting deficits and environmental influences.

Moreover, given that physical dysfunction following TBI can take a myriad of forms and severities, the repertoire of potential interventions required by the TBI therapist is substantial and the skill in applying them appropriately and effectively is complex. In addition, thoughtful attention is demanded by the fact that scientific knowledge is growing exponentially in many fields that have a potential impact on our understanding of the CNS and its functional relationships in both healthy and pathological states.

Therefore, from both practical and theoretical perspectives it can be argued that physiotherapists working in the field of TBI need to have a sufficiently flexible approach to facilitate the application of knowledge from many sources and to allow new learning to be incorporated into practice in a systematic way. By implication, TBI therapists also need to have a wide knowledge base and the ability to assess the value and potential application of emerging evidence.

Since movement is the product of a skeletal and muscular system, driven by central neural mechanisms in response to both routine and changing circumstances, any analytical or problem-solving approach to physical rehabilitation and management needs to embrace all these factors. And, although knowledge is not yet sufficiently advanced to define completely how the physiological systems interact in health or in the presence of neuropathology, a mature model of practice will ultimately reflect a clear understanding of how these systems interrelate and how they may be influenced positively.

Adopting such a framework in principle does not preclude any therapist continuing to use a treatment technique that has been found to be consistently clinically useful but it does require the therapist to entertain the thought that potentially there is another technique, additional element or entirely different approach that may be equally or more effective.

The value of this type of pragmatic approach is recognized by Plant (1998) in her review of 'classic [neuro] physiotherapy approaches' and the theories that underpin them, since she concludes that no existing theoretical model adequately explains motor behaviour. She goes on to highlight the need for physiotherapists to contribute to the development of a future definitive model and in the meantime to rise to the challenge of being selective and innovative in their practice and not to be driven by prescription or dogma.

This is undoubtedly the challenge we face and success can be achieved only through collaboration, open discussion and debate, which in turn requires some basic ground rules and points of facilitation.

ESTABLISHING A COMMON LANGUAGE

On a number of occasions already within this book there has been discussion of the importance of vocabulary and meaning. Discussion and debate is possible only when a common language is used, and it is for this reason that I emphasize the need to minimize the use of ambiguous language or phrases understood only by therapists following a specific treatment approach.

As well as being important in establishing the free flow of ideas and experience across a global audience within physiotherapy, a willingness to adopt vocabulary already in use in the academic literature of other disciplines (and other specialties within our profession) will assist the cross-fertilization required to ensure the development of better theoretical models of motor behaviour in health and disease, and ultimately allow definitive prediction of the best intervention in a particular set of circumstances.

NON-DEFENSIVE STANCE

In addition to considering the use of language, we also have to guard against feelings of threat to our existing practice. It may initially feel that the need to consider change is somehow a criticism of all that has been done before, but this is not the case – and neither is it a constructive response. A more useful viewpoint is to regard reasoned change as positive and developmental, and in practical terms as an *extension* of our potential to help achieve the optimum outcome for the people we work with.

As has already been discussed, without an inclusive theoretical model of motor performance it is not yet possible fully to describe a treatment approach framework or fully explain or defend the interventions we choose to use. However, this is what we need to work towards if we are to be able clearly to describe the rationale for what we do, so that all interested parties can understand, systematically evaluate, confirm or change either the rationale on which a treatment is based or the content of the treatment itself, in the light of new knowledge.

ACKNOWLEDGING PROGRESS AND MOVING ON

The move towards an inclusive treatment approach framework will mean, on the face of it, removing direct reference to long-established approaches and to those pioneering individuals who have contributed enormously to the specialism of neurophysiotherapy. This does not mean leaving behind the knowledge and skills gained as a result of their efforts and in the wider clinical application of their treatment concepts. However, there is a need to establish clarity in our knowledge base without prejudice and this can be done only if all aspects of existing practice are open to scrutiny and can be freely reinterpreted in the light of other evidence.

Already, in practice, the things that differentiate the clinical application of a variety of approaches are diminishing in number. Reflective practitioners from all traditions are increasingly augmenting their core practice with modalities emanating from, or influenced by, other traditions and specialties, as well as by way of a heightened awareness of the literature. This mature eclecticism in practice needs to be better reflected in the stated philosophical basis of clinical practice and this would most honestly be grounded in a model that is openly incomplete and under construction.

If neurophysiotherapists as a whole were to adopt such a working-model approach it would demonstrate the specialty's academic and professional maturity. The confidence that comes with this maturity would allow open admission, for example, that it is not known *how* exactly a particular technique works although it can be demonstrated that its application produces a positive outcome. At the same time, within the same working model, it may well be possible to describe the sound evidential basis for some forms of intervention and tentative explanations for others. With this level of scrutiny it would also be abundantly clear when there is no good reason to continue an aspect of practice that has neither clear clinical benefit nor scientific support.

The working-model approach would therefore allow the inclusion of interventions based on different levels of evidence with the possibility of open evaluation and reclassification as knowledge develops. For example, one classification might be defined as interventions that are developed from established scientific knowledge *and* are proven to be clinically effective. A second could be clinically favoured (though currently scientifically weak) interventions, which ultimately would either disappear to be replaced by a better solution, derived from new knowledge, or would move into the first category described as the scientific evidence for the approach became stronger.

Any attempt to describe such a model in detail across neuropathologies or with reference to all interventions currently in use would result in a hugely complex, confusing, and probably conflicting diagrammatic representation. However, it is feasible, at the present time, for individual practitioners, or groups of practitioners, to apply a set of basic principles which in time and with appropriate evaluation and sharing of data would result in increasing clarity of theory and action.

This process is to some extent already underway with the increasing number of postgraduate researchers from within the profession and the emergence of working groups of researchers coming together from a variety of disciplines to gain a wider perspective in relation to the application of developing knowledge. It would, however, assist both academic progress and effective clinical practice if the process of development were coordinated and there was general awareness of how to contribute to that development.

There is, therefore, a need for agreement on the basic organization and inclusion criteria. This agreement should be brokered across academic and clinical interests, producing an understanding of their reciprocal relationship so that all practitioners accept their role in the evaluation and development of treatment protocols and techniques, and all academic staff and research investigators are willing to explain the potential clinical application of new and developing knowledge. Within such a framework, every practitioner would be able to exercise their professional judgement based on sound knowledge and continue using tried and tested interventions or be innovative as appropriate to the circumstances of their practice.

DEVELOPING AN INCLUSIVE THEORETICAL AND PRACTICE FRAMEWORK

To work towards a framework for theory and practice, practitioners and investigators need to embrace some common principles and adopt consistent standards. A number of factors have already been suggested as being core to this process such as:

- The need for a wide and inclusive knowledge-base (appropriate to the pathology and other specific influencing factors)
- The inclusion of a wide and flexible repertoire of skills and approaches
- The ability at group and individual practitioner level to synthesize and apply appropriate knowledge in defining the approach to intervention, its component parts and the specific content
- Having an inherent evaluative ethos
- Developing explicit mechanisms for the evaluation, discussion and appropriate adoption of new knowledge or new insights.

This or a similar approach is already used and accepted by many individuals who contribute to the practice of neurophysiotherapy but the full benefit will be gained only when it is standard methodology. We will attempt to apply these principles to TBI later in this chapter.

CRITERIA FOR ASSESSING LEVELS OF EVIDENCE

We have already acknowledged that at present the basis of practice differs across practitioners, from mainly anecdotal and clinically based evidence, to an almost exclusive adherence to evidence from published literature. To ensure that no valuable insights are lost, the initial gathering of baseline evidence to develop a framework should aim to be inclusive. However, to allow for evaluation and development from the baseline state, it has to be clear what is known of the clinical value, the theoretical hypothesis or the proven and accepted knowledge of that which is initially included.

In attempting to describe a structure to do this, even for one pathology group, we are reminded immediately of the complexities of physiotherapeutic intervention and why research into clinical practice is often less than straightforward. From the outset it should be recognized that evaluation is not simply about the particular techniques or specific modalities, or the timescale or frequency of an intervention, but also about the context in which it is applied, how it is applied, what else is going on at the time, what has preceded, what is planned to follow, what results are expected, what else may influence those results, and many other potential factors for each individual evaluation.

In order to be clear about the evidence we have and its potential application it may be useful to split the analysis over a number of levels, for example considering separately:

• Manual techniques
• Other modalities or regimes
• The philosophical or behavioural approach used during direct intervention
• The wider theoretical framework from which an approach is drawn, detailing what evidence there is to support each aspect in turn.

The type and source of evidence can also be categorized in terms of clinical effectiveness and scientific bases, for example by considering the applicability of any combination of the following:

• Personal experience of effect (positive or negative, global or specific)
• Clinical consensus of effect (positive or negative, global or specific)
• Theoretical basis (fully developed, partial or newly applied)
• Any applicable or transferable factual information
• Objective evidence of proven use in exactly the circumstances under consideration.

The latter level of evidence, where there is absolute conclusive evidence of positive causal effect of an individual technique or a sequential process, for example, is still rare in neurophysiotherapeutic practice. There are few areas where standardized practice and the theory that underpins that practice are sufficiently developed for both to be tested by way of a randomized controlled trial.

Thus, clinical practice continues to be a dynamic and deductive process that requires a knowledgeable and thinking therapist and as practice already demands a high level of analytical skill, good neurophysiotherapists have a ready ability to apply themselves to the identification and evaluation of the knowledge base. The primary internal barrier seems to be the lack of tradition in, or familiarity with, communication and discussion by way of the written word.

The process just described for categorizing and analysing the evidence may appear unnecessarily complicated, and without direct illustration it is a dry and abstract subject. It is nevertheless important to understand that, until the results of such a wide-ranging evaluation are documented and adopted by neurophysiotherapists as a whole, we cannot expect to achieve consistently high standards of care. Neurophysiotherapy is a complex and challenging area of practice, which will develop as a result of more collaboration across practitioners and between practitioners and researchers. The ultimate aim is to ensure more effective and efficient use of the limited resources available and in so doing to improve the outcome for patients.

PRACTITIONERS' ROLE IN EVALUATION AND DEVELOPMENT

After accepting the need to work towards a common theoretical foundation for practice and the associated prerequisite of agreeing a standard method of analysing the evidence, the final key factor in realizing the goal of best practice lies in understanding the width of responsibility necessary to ensure success. It may appear an obvious statement to say that, in terms of research to improve clinical practice, the clinical therapist has a pivotal role, but this role is not always recognized. Therapists have a responsibility to apply new knowledge within their practice and, just as importantly, they should also be actively involved in defining relevant research questions.

Clinical observations and the questions that arise from the therapeutic interface relate to the whole spectrum of evidence that has just been outlined. For instance, observed patterns in the occurrence of dysfunctional movement over a series of patients can lead to the development of a functionally based hypothesis, the investigation of which may produce a new insight into the course of the associated pathology. Similarly, the application of a treatment, developed from theoretical knowledge, on a case-by-case basis will not only help to establish whether or not it has a positive effect but is also likely to identify factors that are associated with the success or failure in each case.

No matter how well developed the academic theory, the usefulness of the proposed approach, or specific treatment, within everyday practice needs to be evaluated at that level; with real people in real circumstances. The outcome of clinical interventions and the *reasons perceived as central to that outcome* have to inform the acceptance, rejection or further development of the initial theory. This is again dependent on effective communication between clinician, investigator and academic theorist, and a mutual respect and understanding of each for the others' role.

The need for open lines of communication and effective feedback regarding treatment and process outcomes is not confined to the researcher–clinician relationship but is equally relevant as applied to the clinician–clinician relationship. This is particularly important in bridging the gap between the medical model, which is so often the healthcare structure applied in acute provision, and the more pragmatic stance of post-acute services, which necessarily have to allow for the impact of social and personal issues.

No part of the service can operate optimally in isolation and the suggested feedforward and feedback of information outlined in the assessment process (see Chs 4, 5 & 6) applies equally to the evaluation of intervention and the assessment of outcome.

Researchers can assist busy clinicians in a number of ways, for example by producing clearly written analytical review papers and by including more frequent reference to potential clinical applications within reports on primary research projects or, by agreement with the editor, in open letters to be published in the same journal issue.

These examples merely scratch the surface in terms of practical suggestions about how to go about bridging the gap between theory and practice and in developing knowledge of the relationship between the intended outcome of an intervention and the actual result. The effective solution will differ with respect to the *local application* of establishing working clinical and academic links.

However, the importance of the principle of ensuring effective communication and the acceptance of mutual responsibility and ownership of the evaluative process cannot be stressed enough and, similarly, the primary need for communication to be effective across the profession. The primary message is that everyone has a responsibility to contribute to the knowledge base either by direct research or by engaging in evaluative discussion.

DEVELOPING A WORKING MODEL FOR TBI INTERVENTIONS

Potential physiotherapeutic interventions following TBI, as has already been stated, are vast in number because of the variety in severity, mix of deficit, venue of contact, time since the primary injury, functional goals and other influencing factors. It is not sufficient, in an attempt to introduce clarity to the process, simply to break the analysis down into acute, sub-acute and post-acute interventions as this would not deal adequately with the range of severity or the influence of a functional goal, for example.

However, although this difficulty in clearly categorizing people who have sustained a TBI into neat groupings may initially appear to be an additional complication, it does help avoid the temptation to become prescriptive. The examples outlined in the remainder of this chapter should, therefore, be regarded as just that: examples of deficit profiles that may be found following TBI and examples of some of the literature that may be considered as part of the decision-making process that is the foundation of reflective clinical practice.

FOUNDATIONS FOR PRACTICE

We have outlined a basic working-model structure as a philosophical approach to achieving practice based on evidence. Before going on to illustrate the application of that approach in a variety of circumstances after TBI, we will first review the basic foundations on which present-day neurorehabilitation is based.

There are essentially two related principles derived from current knowledge and emerging evidence. The first is that human beings are living, changing organisms, capable of significant adaptation to meet changing demands. That is, even though in the adult some aspects of our structure tends to remain constant, for example the length of the long bones after epiphyseal fusion, other structures and processes routinely adapt and change in response to new or changing demands. Clinically, this can be seen, for example, in muscle bulk changes following training and it is also known that other internal changes occur in response to repetitive physical (Karni et al 1995, Moritatani & deVries 1979, Nadler et al 1998) and cognitive (Karni & Bertini 1997, Kopelman et al 1998) demands.

In addition, it is known that particular biochemical and structural changes are associated with the relative frequency and persistence of the new demand, with neural facilitation in the main preceding structural change (Kidd et al 1992). This inherent adaptive ability, as applied to the structure and functions of immediate concern to neurophysiotherapists, is sometimes referred to as neuromuscular plasticity, emphasizing that the potential for structural and functional change applies to both the peripheral muscular system and the internal workings of the CNS.

The second principle is that the same mechanisms and inherent abilities remain viable following injury or other pathological events. There is clearly a need to allow for the impact of actual tissue loss, and the site and extent of any permanent damage will affect the organism's capability to recover, but the remaining healthy tissue should retain at least the same inherent properties as before. If this assumption is indeed the case, there are several implications that follow, such as:

- The changes that are enforced on the human organism as a result of the pathological event(s) may themselves lead to internal biochemical and structural change

- The preservation or reintroduction of normal experience should help promote internal structural normality
- Inactivity is not a neutral state in terms of the basic maintenance of structure and function
- There is no predestined functional outcome of any neural pathology.

The latter point is supported by a number of studies illustrating that the nature of the observed adaptation is task and/or context dependent (for a review see Carr & Shepherd 1998), emphasizing the potential for postinjury management and rehabilitative intervention to contribute either positively or negatively to any reorganization that takes place. Similarly, habitual placement in, or adoption of, malaligned postures and/or repetitive practice of compensatory movement strategies may be expected to facilitate or reinforce internal changes that will potentiate their subsequent reproduction.

Although a number of mechanisms, including axonal sprouting and various modifications in synaptic connections, have been identified as having the potential to replace or compensate for lost neural tissue, research in this area is still in the exploratory phase. There is, however, huge potential in this regard for the effects of physiotherapeutic treatment to be evaluated using modern imaging methods such as positron emission tomography (PET), functional magnetic resonance imaging (fMRI) and transcranial magnetic stimulation (TMS) first to identify a change in CNS activity and subsequently for any lasting change to be understood in terms of structural adaptation.

Returning to the application of knowledge of plasticity in preserved tissue, neurophysiotherapists might reasonably adopt a similar maxim to our medical colleagues who swear to 'do no harm', by striving first to allow no additional harm to befall their patients in terms of secondary negative neuromuscular plasticity. Achieving such a treatment goal would also ensure the optimal starting point for any further reorganization or relearning that can subsequently be induced.

This principle of maintaining the integrity of soft tissue and therefore the optimum potential for function is, of course, easily recognizable as a core principle of teaching throughout the history of the physiotherapy profession, which developed from the clinical observation of the negative results of failing to do so well in advance of any supportive scientific evidence. Within neurorehabilitation, however, this principle was in the main applied only to those in a paralysed or unconscious state, and traditionally comprised a regime of passive or passive-assisted stretches to try to maintain range of motion.

This type of intervention was found clinically to be of limited use in the management of patients with severely heightened tonal states, such as in acute severe TBI or in severe complex neurodisability. Subsequently, the use of casting and early weight-bearing was introduced in an effort to manage better the immediate and severe physical consequences of decerebrate and decorticate posturing caused by severe TBI. Similarly, Pope (1992), working within the principle of managing the overall condition rather than simply treating symptoms or impairments, highlighted the importance of active positional control (throughout day and night) in preventing further physical deterioration in the presence of neuropathology.

In a parallel development, which would seem to support primary intervention targeted at maintaining the integrity of the musculoskeletal system, recent evidence has suggested that the resistance to passive movement interpreted by clinicians as spasticity of neural origin may be caused by both neural mechanisms, such as increased stretch reflex excitability, *and* by changes in the mechanical and elastic properties of the muscle (Berger et al 1984, Carey & Burghardt 1993, Dietz et al 1981, Thilman et al 1991). Some authors go as far as to consider that the development of spasticity secondary to neuropathology may, in part, *be potentiated* by the presence of contracture (Brown 1994, O'Dwyer et al 1996).

It has also been suggested that some of the physical characteristics of Parkinson disease represent secondary adaptive compensations rather than a single primary lesion-specific movement disorder, and similarly that the disordered movement characteristics of Down's syndrome may develop as a result of cognitive limitations (Latash 1993).

It would seem, therefore, that the genesis of what may previously have been regarded as primary neural impairments or direct symptoms of neural injury or disease may be influenced by a greater number of factors. If the development of neurodisability is such a fluid and interactive process, it follows that there is significantly more potential to influence the functional outcome than has previously been recognized.

It is therefore imperative to consider the origins and presence of, or the potential for, a wide range of adaptive changes and/or compensatory mechanisms in the neuromuscular system, or in how it is used functionally, as part of the physical assessment process. It also follows that it is necessary to include proactive management of potential negative changes in the design of any planned intervention.

When the presence of adaptive changes is recognized, further analysis is then required in order to try to identify the pathological, behavioural and environmental factors that have combined to produce the presenting physical status. If causal factors can be identified, then the information may be used in treatment planning for the individual concerned and potentially to prevent similar developments in subsequent cases.

Furthermore, the scope of any planned intervention, and the expected outcome, can be informed by an assessment of whether or not the adaptations or compensations seen represent the optimum solution to the underlying movement disorder. Consideration should also be given to the question of whether or not the current movement habit is likely to limit the potential for further functional recovery or even fuel a negative spiral of diminishing function.

Thus, to achieve the goal of evidence-based, or even knowledge-informed, neurophysiotherapeutic practice we must systematically gather and document the pathophysiological and environmental influences in each case, state the hypotheses on which interventions are based, and record the outcomes with analysis of facilitative and/or confounding factors. We should be able to share our successes and failures, confident in the knowledge that no-one has all the answers and that we all have some of the insights. In this way we cannot fail to develop further our understanding of the true genesis and development of neurodisability and therefore identify all the parameters that need to be addressed by the whole rehabilitation team.

EXAMPLES OF WORKING MODELS

Each of the examples given below follows a consistent approach to describing a working model based on the principles previously outlined. First, an initial decision is made regarding what core subject areas or factors are appropriate to include in the knowledge base that will then be used to inform practice. Second, current treatment approaches and techniques are listed. Third, an attempt is made to identify links between published evidence and practice, and/or to document other reasoned arguments as to why that particular aspect of practice should or should not continue to be included.

From this process, in each example a series of statements and questions emerges that represents a partial evaluation of current knowledge with regard to the particular area. Clearly, the examples in no way reflect *all* practice and the conclusions cannot be regarded as complete. However, the intention is simply to illustrate a process that all therapists can adopt to examine their own practice while at the same time addressing some clinically relevant issues.

Additional examples of programme design, content and delivery are outlined in the following chapter.

AN EXAMPLE WORKING MODEL FOR ACUTE SEVERE TBI

This example applies the working-model approach to physiotherapeutic intervention within the first 2 weeks for someone who has sustained a closed TBI resulting in an extended period of deep unconsciousness. In this example the injured person has no additional skeletal or internal injuries.

Primary evidence base

The following list is suggested as a starting point for the scope of knowledge required to inform physiotherapeutic practice for this subgroup of patients:

- Pathophysiology of TBI (including relevant risk factors)
- Principles of acute medical management
- Physiotherapy role in achieving medical management goals
- Appropriate respiratory literature
- Anatomy, physiology and neuromuscular knowledge (including theories of plasticity)
- TBI outcome studies, known deficit profiles
- Methods of preventing or limiting deficits (controlling risk factors)
- Psychosocial consequences of stress and loss

Common treatment goals and approaches

This list outlines some principles of treatment and goal specific interventions commonly targeted in this subgroup of patients:

1. Continuous assessment
2. Intervention and management strategies to promote optimum blood oxygenation
3. Positioning, assisted movement and casting (proactive, reactive) to preserve the integrity of soft tissues, skin and range of motion
4. Sensory stimulation
5. Provision of information and education for family and friends
6. Use of frequent, short treatments with the gradual reintroduction of antigravity positioning and the experience of movement.

Discussion

There is a full literature with regard to the pathophysiology of TBI and medical management principles within acute care (see Ch. 2). There are three main areas of direct relevance to the physiotherapist. The first relates to respiratory and cardiovascular health, which is covered in some depth in Chapter 2, the second to musculoskeletal integrity, and the third to level of awareness.

Respiratory and cardiovascular health

Optimum respiratory function is central in limiting secondary cerebral damage and in stabilizing the overall condition. However, the presence of raised intracranial pressure (ICP), or the patient's susceptibility to developing raised ICP, are factors indicating caution in the choice of physical intervention to achieve that goal. Specifically this means avoiding or minimizing events that raise ICP and balancing the aggressiveness of intervention with the needs of each individual case.

This clinical decision-making process, along with discussion and description of the interventions of choice in a variety of respiratory circumstances, has been clearly described by Ada and colleagues (1990). This information, presented within an evidence-based chapter on the physiotherapeutic care of the unconscious TBI patient, is a synthesis of the respiratory literature, pathophysiological knowledge of TBI and extensive clinical experience, making clear links between much of the evidence base and treatment goal 2.

It is of particular note that, in contrast to a number of other interventions and positioning manoeuvres associated with standard respiratory care, percussion, performed with a slow single-hand action, has been found to lower ICP (Garrad & Bullock 1986, Paratz & Burns 1993).

Musculoskeletal integrity and neuromuscular status

Published literature highlights the frequent presence of immediate, gross hypertonic states and also the potential for significant residual physical deficits following severe TBI, beyond lack of or impaired volitional movement, such as contracture, spasticity and tissue breakdown, for example (Collin & Daly 1998, Hillier et al 1997, Rusk et al 1966). Specific additional risks are also highlighted such as heterotopic ossification, particularly in adolescents and in the presence of multiple fractures (Citta-Pietrolungo et al 1992, Hurvitz et al 1992).

In terms of managing negative physical manifestations, there are direct reports relating to specific early management intervention (casting and prolonged stretch) designed to limit the development of soft tissue adaptation and loss of range following TBI (Bernard et al 1984, Conine et al 1990, Sullivan et al 1988) or to reverse early observed changes (Booth et al 1983, Cornall 1992, Mills 1984, Moseley 1997). All of these reports support in general the principles of preventing or reversing the structural changes in soft tissues known to occur as a result of immobilization (Goldspink & Williams 1990), and are primarily concerned with methods of controlling the imbalance in muscle resting length resultant from the hypertonic states.

However, although some authors recommend early proactive casting for the prevention of foot and ankle deformity (Conine et al 1990, Edwards & Charlton 1996), a position that is supported by clinical experience in the case of severe injuries, the details of specific inclusion criteria and optimum length of application for these casts or for others used later in the physical management programme have yet to be defined. Similarly, anticipated problems of bony demineralization (McLellan 1993) and threats to periarticular structures (Akeson et al 1980) are incorporated into the wider rationale of routinely including weight-bearing and movement within the management approach (with appropriate measures to ensure cardiovascular and ICP stability).

Comparative studies in these areas have not yet been undertaken but it is worthy of note that, contrary to a frequently rehearsed argument against casting, pressure area problems or tissue breakdown were not identified as complications in any of the reported studies. All casts were applied following a strict protocol.

The principles of neuroplasticity are also being applied when using assisted movement into a normal range of basic antigravity positions such as supported sitting and supported standing, with the aim of achieving normal biomechanical alignment and sensory experience (see below).

Clinically, the inclusion of routine lower limb casting in severe TBI and early movement into supported antigravity positions in acute care has produced an improvement in physical outcome as measured by physical status on entry to an outpatient programme, both in terms of improved extensibility of the posterior tibials and diminished upper trunk extensor tone (personal observation).

Level of awareness

The impact on the damaged brain, via the whole of the individual's sensory systems, of all episodes of physical contact and communication, as well as their ongoing awareness of the surrounding environment, needs to be considered in agreeing the general management approach, as well as in the choice of specific treatment techniques. Principles can be derived with reference to the pathophysiology of TBI, the limitations of sensory processing in the damaged brain, the neurophysiological processes that underpin the concept of plasticity and the knowledge of heightened neural excitability in the immediate postinjury period.

Pertinent aspects of sensory processing and inferred limitations in the presence of brain injury are reviewed by Wood (1991), with particular reference to sensory stimulation programmes for individuals in the vegetative state, but the cautionary emphasis inherent in this article is equally appropriate in the immediate postinjury period when the metabolic and electrical function of the brain is destabilized, and later in the recovery process when the danger of sensory saturation remains (Gandevia & Burke 1984). Ada and colleagues (1990, p. 279) describe their favoured approach in terms of 'ensuring the patient receives a normal amount of sensory input, both auditory and visual, rather than by using methods that rely on overloading the person with non-specific sensory input'.

To achieve this in a busy ward environment might reasonably include the use of eye guards or ear protectors, the application of which may have an impact on the later incidence of auditory or visual hypersensitivity, which can be disabling long-term deficits.

As well as being appropriate to respiratory health in this type of patient, a treatment strategy of high-frequency review and short intervention time is consistent with balancing the desire to facilitate a range of positions, movements and normal sensory experiences with the caution not to over-stimulate or overexcite the damaged brain or fail to allow adequate rest and recovery.

Finally, all aspects of pathology-related knowledge, combined with knowledge of the psychosocial impact of the traumatic event on those who are close to the injured individual, will allow appropriate presentation of information to relatives and friends, and a degree of understanding of their experience (see Ch. 3).

Resultant issues

Much of the management and intervention strategy outlined in this example is supported by evidence, at least at the level of developing a theoretical rationale from basic science. Clinically based research is required to test those theories and to provide comparative information on the efficacy of individual treatment components and, for example, the utility of different materials for casting.

AN EXAMPLE WORKING MODEL FOR ACUTE MODERATE TBI

This example applies the working-model approach to physiotherapeutic intervention within a short acute period of contact with an adolescent male who sustained a TBI resulting in a period of unconsciousness of less than 2 hours and who has throughout continued to breath spontaneously. The injured young man also has a left femoral fracture and an undisplaced pelvic fracture, which are seen as the primary issue of medical concern. Consciousness was regained in the emergency department, the femoral fracture fixed internally and aftercare is being provided on an orthopaedic ward.

Primary evidence base

- Pathophysiology of TBI and skeletal fractures (including relevant risk factors)
- Principles of acute medical management (TBI and orthopaedic)
- Physiotherapy role in achieving medical management goals
- Anatomy, physiology and neuromuscular knowledge (including theories of plasticity)

- TBI outcome studies, known deficit profiles
- Psychosocial consequences of stress and loss
- Principles of the management of patients with cognitive dysfunction
- Principles and practice of early rehabilitation (TBI and orthopaedic)

Common treatment goals and approaches

1. Primary and ongoing assessment
2. Monitor respiratory function, promote optimum blood oxygenation
3. Position, use active, assisted movement and casting (proactive or reactive) to preserve the integrity of soft tissues, skin and range of motion
4. Use active intervention within the limits of the effects of the TBI
5. Mobilize within the limits defined by the orthopaedic surgeon
6. Orientate and reassure
7. Inform and educate the individual, the family and friends
8. Provide education for colleagues
9. Ensure onward referral.

Discussion

As in the first example, physiotherapeutic intervention in relation to this case is initially concerned with cardiovascular and respiratory health, and with musculoskeletal integrity In addition, as the individual is functioning at a higher level of awareness, consideration is given to the promotion of skills for functional independence. Finally, an indirect educational role may be indicated with relatives and friends, and with colleagues inexperienced in dealing with the sequelae of CNS damage (see Ch. 4).

Respiratory and cardiovascular health

Maintenance of a good oxygenated blood supply is crucial to the ideal of promoting optimal conditions for healing and recovery. Inspired oxygen is recommended to meet the brain's increased requirements (Frost 1985) and it should be humidified to limit the drying action of the oxygen (Ada et al 1990).

Neurological depression of respiratory function, abnormal breathing patterns, immobility, increased risk of infection and local injury are all potential threats to the respiratory system (Ellis 1990) and, in addition, this patient has also undergone surgery under anaesthesia, which can depress normal mechanisms for maintaining respiratory health (Lunn 1991).

Close liaison with medical and nursing staff will be required to achieve a good balance in pain control to minimize the inhibitory effect on respiratory function of pain from the pelvic damage, without further compromising respiratory drive. The combination of injuries carries a risk of deep vein thrombosis and fat embolus, and indicates the need for vigilance in case of any sudden change in the patient's condition. Any immobilization should be kept to a minimum.

Musculoskeletal integrity and neuromuscular status

The patient's age raises the possibility of heterotopic ossification (HO), although the relatively short duration of coma probably decreases that risk (Hurvitz et al 1992). Anecdotally, *aggressive* physical intervention to increase or maintain range of motion in the presence of hypertonicity is said to contribute to the development of HO, but there is no direct evidence to support this theory in the TBI population.

Commonly, bone healing in the presence of TBI is accelerated and bone salts may be laid down in damaged muscle, particularly adjacent to bone fractures. HO may simply occur as a result of central neural factors independent of management factors.

My own experience of symptomatic HO after TBI has been predominantly in cases where prolonged immobility has occurred, as in a case of a boy with decerebrate posturing, who had not been actively treated and had remained in coma for several years, or in several patients with more moderate injuries with femoral and/or tibial fractures who were immobilized in bed on traction.

It is interesting to note that in a prospective study of 111 young patients with TBI (aged 6–21 years) involving bone scanning within 3 weeks of admission, 25 were found to have HO at a point when only two had clinical signs. Ten patients remained clinically asymptomatic. All patients diagnosed with HO received 'aggressive ROM (*range of movement*) by physical and occupational therapy' and only three patients had decreased range and/or discomfort at discharge (Citta-Pietrolungo et al 1992). The therapeutic intervention used in this study was not detailed and long-term follow-up was not reported.

Gross hypertonic postures are not a management problem in this case example, and therefore casting is not indicated. However, physical assessment reveals apparently decreased muscular tone without loss of ability to initiate movement in the three limbs that can easily be handled.

There is poor limb–girdle stability, and initial difficulty achieving and sustaining unsupported sitting. There is also distress on first attempts at supported standing, with fear of falling rather than pain being perceived as the reason. Repeated eye closure is also noted during these procedures. The patient is not distressed in supine or supported long-sitting in bed.

All these factors suggest some midline cerebellar involvement. Without active intervention the orthopaedic, motor and sensory problems have the potential to reinforce the negative functional effects resultant from each individual problem.

Promotion of skills for functional independence

The difficulty in achieving and maintaining basic antigravity positions has clear implications for regaining functional independence, particularly in the presence of some visual dysfunction. Although it is very early in the process of recovery, these factors indicate that the period of physical recovery will be extended beyond the period that would be a normal length of stay taking into account the orthopaedic injuries alone. The presence of specific neural symptoms may also be a marker to indicate more widespread cerebral damage (see Ch. 2).

In these circumstances an appropriate specialized inpatient rehabilitation placement should be sought as a matter of priority. Meanwhile, assistance and advice should be obtained from available colleagues in other disciplines and/or a physiotherapist with specialist knowledge to supplement any basic knowledge of cognitive dysfunction and the immediate assessment findings based on structured observation of behaviours.

The processing limitations of the damaged brain outlined in the previous example continue to apply, and the demands of taking part in self-care tasks should not be underestimated. Combining neuromuscular goals with care tasks, and agreeing a paced and graded series of interventions with occupational therapy and nursing colleagues in particular, will help to avoid excessive demands without promoting inactivity.

Educative and facilitative role

The acute nature of the injury, the need to pace interventions and the patient's apparent distress during attempts to adopt antigravity positions will limit the length of treatment sessions. The reasoning behind the intervention approach can be explained to both the injured person and their family, and should be based on knowledge of pathology, time course and anticipated outcome. When the level of cognition has not been formally assessed, it is appropriate to adopt a cautious estimate of how much is being retained from contact to contact.

Simple explanation and re-explanation of the individual's circumstances and each part of the planned intervention can be included as a matter of routine, allowing anticipation of, and preparation for, potentially distressing sensations such as dizziness or blurred vision. The need to work through the dizziness in a *controlled* way to drive the recovery process may not be easily understood and will probably run contrary to the instinct of patient, family and inexperienced staff alike. Issues such as this, if not discussed overtly, have the potential to undermine relationships, trust and functional outcome.

Families value explanation of the factors influencing the chosen interventions, and clearly reasoned explanations will reassure and open lines of communication so that issues of concern are heard. As described in Chapter 3, this is the beginning of a lengthy journey for friends and family as well as the injured individual, and the provision of immediate and ongoing accurate information and support is key to the long-term health of the patient's support structure.

In some areas a specific service for carers may be available within health or social care provision as well as via self-help groups and campaigning organizations. The important point is that appropriate referrals are made and/or contact information is given so that families are in the best position to make informed decisions about onward placement, home discharge and related issues.

Resultant issues

In considering this second example, evidence is available to direct and support the principles of primary management and in gauging (mainly medical) risk factors. Beyond this, intervention and management plans are based mostly on applied knowledge of long-term sequelae of TBI, some neurophysiological processes and limited evidence of the superiority of specialist teams over uncoordinated provision by non-specialist clinicians. Consensus guidance from experienced TBI practitioners is, at present, still based primarily on what we know has failed individuals with TBI, and their families, in the past rather than what has been specifically proven to work via formal research.

It is, however, important to acknowledge the level of agreement on basic principles that exists worldwide across experienced TBI practitioners and also to emphasize the role that feedback and insights from carers and TBI survivors has played in shaping some of the basic principles. It may make practical and economic sense to adopt these commonly supported, though unproven, assumptions so that the research agenda can move forward to address the value of specific interventions in parallel with current and developing clinical practice.

This and the previous example both address physiotherapeutic provision within acute care and presume that care will be delivered within a medical model. The final example of applying a structured approach to identifying what, if any, evidence there is to support current practice looks at post-acute provision within a rehabilitation ethos.

AN EXAMPLE WORKING MODEL FOR POST-ACUTE SEVERE TBI

This example applies the working-model approach to physiotherapeutic intervention in the case of a 20-year-old woman who sustained a TBI resulting in 12 days of deep coma and a post-traumatic amnesia of almost 2 months. She is now 16 months' postinjury. She had no bony injuries but has occasional oedema of the right knee.

The woman began a staged discharge from inpatient provision at 10 months' postinjury and was a day patient (initially 5 days per week, reducing to 2 days) between months 12 and 14. There has been a 6-week break from therapy before commencing an outpatient programme 2 weeks ago.

Primary evidence base

- Pathophysiology of TBI, soft tissue injury
- Anatomy, physiology and neuromuscular knowledge (including biomechanics, motor performance and plasticity)
- TBI rehabilitation programmes, outcome studies, known deficit profiles
- Psychosocial consequences of stress and loss
- Neurorehabilitation theories and treatment approaches
- Motor skill acquisition
- Principles of, and treatment approaches in, the management of patients with cognitive dysfunction
- Psychosocial rehabilitation

Common treatment goals and approaches

1. Initial and ongoing assessment
2. Reduce or eliminate factors having a negative influence on motor performance
3. Maximize the experience of normal motor performance
4. Maximize the integrity and/or performance of physical structures upon which motor performance is dependent
5. Maximize the performance of functional movement
6. Maximize the performance of component parts of functional movement
7. Maximize activity levels, achieve functional goals
8. Use facilitation techniques
9. Use inhibitory techniques
10. Use guided training
11. Use unsupervised training
12. Emphasize real-life activities

13. Provide information and education for the individual and for family and friends
14. Provide education for colleagues
15. Access and apply knowledge from colleagues.

Discussion

This example, beyond the principles of early management associated with the first two examples, is altogether more complex but it is indicative of the scope of intervention and diversity within existing clinical practice. Items from the list of goals and approaches given above would certainly be found in an audit of various therapeutic notes relating to cases similar to that described above, and the list is by no means complete.

It may be considered that the extent and diversity of the content is made necessary by the fact that the basic information given in this case example is non-specific in terms of sensorimotor findings. It could also be said that treatment goals and the appropriate approach would be more easily described given a more detailed case outline, and this would be a reasonable assertion.

However, I would like to use the limited description of physical deficits within this final example as a vehicle to re-emphasize the importance of the interrelationship between the physical assessment and the rest of the global assessment. I would also like to open the discussion of evidence to include reference to a wider range of clinically relevant issues and associated literature than would be possible within the confines of one, or even several, rehabilitation case examples.

After focusing on physical issues it seems important to stop and reiterate the importance of considering factors other than immediate physical signs in planning relevant and feasible interventions. In post-acute TBI physical rehabilitation, the identification of the appropriate treatment goals and therapeutic approach and the prediction of a realistic outcome are highly dependent on much more than the physical deficits. This is also probably true for the majority of rehabilitation programmes, and in Chapter 4 I have already argued that the consideration of other factors should be explicit in determining the scope of intervention for physiotherapists within any TBI service.

However, in acute care, as in our two previous examples, many of the same influencing factors are controlled by the process of achieving medical stability and/or by the structure of the hospital environment. It is only when these management and physical structures are removed that the impact of non-physical factors is increasingly observed and arguably becomes more important to consider.

In this chapter I have been advancing an argument for each practitioner to identify and evaluate evidence to support or refute physical interventions and methods of physical management, and I have suggested a process template for doing so. Although it is imperative that physiotherapists develop an informed understanding of issues pertinent to physical matters and have a strong rationale for their interventions, functional success cannot be achieved in a physical vacuum.

It remains crucial to a holistic approach to understand that the answers to the questions of what goal is realistic, what treatment approach and/or techniques are appropriate, and what outcome might be expected of that intervention cannot be derived simply from analysis of physical symptoms. We will, therefore, consider the impact of cognitive function and lifestyle preferences on the design, delivery and expectations of physical intervention in the next chapter.

The second reason for choosing not to describe this young woman's physical status in detail takes us full circle to the issues discussed at the beginning of the chapter. The lack of a complete theory of motor performance, our incomplete knowledge of the effects of neuropathology on motor performance, the inconsistencies and conflicting philosophies underpinning clinical practice, and the use of exclusive vocabulary by some practitioners, all make the task of describing a complete and accurate picture of physical status in writing very difficult indeed. What would be understood as a primary or secondary impairment, what would be regarded as a compensation, and what vocabulary would be necessary to impart a clear picture of the physical presentation, at this time remains largely a function of the therapist's philosophical approach.

To move beyond these difficulties we have to devise a working-model framework capable of describing current knowledge independently of conceptual approach and we have to demonstrate the ability to develop that framework further on a sound evidential basis. I will conclude this chapter with brief reference to some of the studies and published literature that I believe should be included in our thinking in the process of developing knowledge-informed and clinically effective practice.

CONSIDERATIONS IN DEVELOPING A THEORETICAL FRAMEWORK

This review is brief and selective, and is designed primarily to encourage thought. No specific conclusions are offered but I hope readers will be intrigued enough to read more, to develop and/or test treatment hypotheses, and to share the results with us all.

Many of the examples given relate to developing knowledge of structure and function in the absence of pathology. I accept the basic argument that this does not automatically relate to action and response in the presence of pathology. None the less, I would argue that it is imperative to understand what the range of normal is if we are to continue to assess motor performance against expected normal and to base our therapeutic goals around achieving motor performance that approximates to normal.

BASIC STRUCTURE AND FUNCTION

Muscles

Muscles have a number of inherent qualities, some of which are dependent on the muscle fibre composition and/or the functional role that the individual muscles play. All muscles are said to possess spring-like attributes, that is, they have a tendency to resist stretch. However, muscles are more complex than simple springs in that their length–tension relationship is curved and not linear, and they also have a dynamic component of stiffness such that there is additional resistance to stretch *during the lengthening process* which disappears when the muscle stops lengthening (Gordon 1990).

The inherent tension in muscle from a biomechanical point of view, therefore, has both an elastic and a dynamic component so that the perception of stiffness in a muscle will be different depending on the length of the muscle (and how this relates to the resting length) and the speed at which the muscle is being lengthened. The resting length of a muscle is dependent on its internal structure, its current functional use and its current relationship with the CNS. All three of these factors are open to change and are interrelated.

For convenience of discussion, muscle structure is frequently separated into contractile and non-contractile components. We have already acknowledged a number of structural changes that are associated with immobilization and disuse, such as atrophy, length changes and increased collagen : muscle fibre ratio. We know that, experimentally, the type and extent of these (and other) structural changes may be influenced by extrinsic factors, such as positioning, stretch, activity and diet (Goldspink and Williams 1990). We also know that there is a two-way relationship between the structure of muscle and the performance required of it in routine function. This is exemplified by the potential for change in basic muscle fibre composition.

Put simply, the contractile component of muscles contains, in varying ratios, muscle fibres that either respond slowly and are slow to fatigue (type I), respond quickly and fatigue easily (type IIa), or respond quickly but fatigue less quickly than type IIa (type IIb). Postural muscles, for example, contain predominantly type I fibres. The type of muscle fibre is initially determined by the motor neurone that innervates the muscle unit to which it belongs (Vrbova et al 1978), but changes in the functional use (including inactivity) of the muscle within which the muscle unit is contained can induce fibre-type changes (Pette and Vrbova 1985).

There are enormous implications for therapeutic assessment and rehabilitation practice of the fact that changes in muscle use can induce structural changes that impact on subsequent muscle performance. It is particularly pertinent that changes can occur without any primary contribution from CNS factors, that is, in the absence of CNS pathology.

There are implications both for movement habits adopted by patients and for compensation strategies taught by rehabilitation professionals alike.

For example, patients who habitually use the upper limbs for postural support can anticipate a decrease in the speed of response of those muscles, possibly affecting dexterity or even the ability to use saving reactions. Similarly, regaining any motor skill or functional activity that requires muscles to work at either end of the spectrum (either quick response or sustained activity) demands rehabilitative activities that include repetitive practice of exactly the type of activity that is required.

This potential for change in muscle structure and function *in the absence of primary neuropathology* is clearly of relevance in our re-examination of muscle tone, and particularly in the quest to understand exactly what spasticity is.

Neural connections

Looking beyond muscle, there is interesting emergent evidence in relation to local, spinal and central neural connections. Earlier in this chapter we discussed the fact that many physiotherapy techniques have focused on the manipulation of the *peripheral* musculoskeletal system because it is visible and tangible, and because clinical changes have been observed in response to some of these interventions. The presumption has been that this peripheral input somehow mediates internal change, and a number of specific hypotheses in this regard have been advanced to explain both treatment approaches and observed change.

Much remains to be proven or dismissed in this area but a growing number of standardized methods of investigation of reflexes, muscular activity and the role of different afferent inputs now offer the opportunity to look at immediate reactions and longer term changes in response to a variety of peripheral manipulations.

Similarly, there is now the technology to determine exactly which parts of the system become dysfunctional as a result of a particular neuropathology. Taken together, a baseline measure of *internal* dysfunction and the ability to measure any change during or following an intervention would seem to hold tremendous promise for evaluation and improvement of treatment techniques.

Clinicians, of course, do not have immediate access to scanners, electromyography or transcranial stimulators but we can access the results of laboratory studies in journals such as *Brain, Experimental Brain Research, Neuromuscular Disorders* or *Disability and Rehabilitation*, to name only a few, or in summary form in publications like *Current Opinion in Neurology*. In addition, as a number of laboratory techniques become more portable, we need to be linking up with those who have the technological know-how to take studies beyond the present focus on normal function or the limitations of laboratory-based tasks.

Reflex pathways, muscle recruitment and fatigue, similarities and differences in sensing and action and many other facets of central–peripheral interaction are, individually, specialist areas of study. Each aspect of investigation is specialized in terms of methods of investigation and in its own body of literature, and I would not begin to claim in-depth knowledge in any of these areas. As an example, however, I will describe one area that I believe has potential clinical significance and that would benefit from further thought and investigation.

There are a number of lines of enquiry that would seem to suggest that the control and performance of movement of the forearm and hand is quite different from that in other body parts. This inference is drawn from documented differences in the role of sensory nerve endings (Gandevia et al 1992), differences in reflex pathways (Dietz 1995) and differences in the size of direct cortical connections (Lemon 1995).

The primary message at this time would seem to be that skilled manipulation is highly dependent on intact cortical function and intact (two-way) fast connections between the structures of the distal arm and the cortex. It may be that this offers some explanation as to why dexterity remains a problem for some patients who make an otherwise good physical recovery.

Clinically, it would seem important to remember this knowledge when planning interventions and, in particular, to consider whether it might be reasonable to adopt a different approach to rehabilitation for manual skills as compared to when addressing gait or balance.

It may be reasonable to consider that specific treatment techniques that are thought to work via spinal connections may not be effective in re-educating hand skills. Conversely, skill acquisition theories developed and tested predominantly via upper limb studies may not be directly applicable to gait. Nothing is certain in the immediate practical application of this type of information but it does provide a focus for reflection on current and past practice and suggests questions for formal study.

Location-specific functions

Another expanding area of current study that has significant potential to inform neurophysiotherapeutic practice is the identification of differential areas of brain activity during a variety of physical and other functional tasks. The choice of treatment approach and eventually predictions of outcome will be assisted by specific knowledge of damaged areas combined with the type of dysfunction associated with those areas. This is of particular relevance to rehabilitation after TBI given the diffuse and complex nature of injuries.

Again this is a large area of study and it is possible to give only a few brief highlights but, as in the preceding example relating to the importance of cortical connections for manipulative skills, there is significant food for thought in the exploration of how to apply and test this new knowledge for practical therapeutic effect.

Studies suggest that specific locations may take a lead role for aspects of motor performance within a distributed processing model. For example, Jueptner and Weiller (1998) have recently undertaken a review to try to differentiate the role of the basal ganglia from that of the cerebellum during movement.

Based on recent functional imaging work with humans, and with reference to previous animal studies, they propose that the basal ganglia is concerned with selecting appropriate movements or selecting appropriate muscles to perform a movement already selected by the premotor cortex. In contrast, they assert that the neocerebellum is involved in monitoring and optimizing movements using sensory feedback. Moreover, they state that between 80% and 90% of cerebellar activity during the performance of some motor tasks is attributable to sensory processing, while the basal ganglia are not involved at all in sensory processing.

Schluter and colleagues (1998) also identify the premotor cortex as important in the selection of movements (after a visual cue) and suggest that there is left hemisphere dominance for rapid selection of action. Other work has suggested that the premotor cortex is more likely to be involved in the selection of movement in response to an external stimulus, whereas the supplementary motor area is more concerned with internally generated movements (Passingham 1987).

More recently a variety of studies has revealed differences in activation depending on the type, complexity and length of the task used, including activation of parts of the posterior parietal lobe during motor selection with auditory as well as visual cues (Dieber et al 1991, Grafton et al 1992).

While, on one level, this information may be regarded as confusing, it does emphasize the complexity of the process of selection of movement appropriate to stimulus; it also highlights the distributed nature of accessing stored motor programmes and, possibly, offers potential for teaching compensatory strategies where one part of the selection system is dysfunctional.

Vision and task-oriented movement

One of the major criticisms I would level at my own past practice would be the limited way in which I have *consciously* used vision within rehabilitation programmes and/or considered visual dysfunction within the analysis of functional performance. The visual and proprioceptive systems (including the vestibular system) are key to the successful orientation of the body within the external environment and to the appropriate organization of body segments for the task in hand (Shumway-Cook and Woollacott 1995). These sensory modalities are also central to the monitoring and effective execution of movement required for each motor task.

More than one third of the human brain is involved with the recognition and processing of visual information (Stein 1995). Not all visual information is used *directly* to guide eye and limb movement but much of the visual system does play a part, for example appropriate object recognition is important in the process of judging the grip and force required to lift a particular object.

The posterior parietal cortex (PPC) appears to coordinate a distributed neural network which can target attention, move the eyes, body and limbs appropriate to the task and the environment (Stein 1992). Damage to the PPC itself or to any of the functionally linked areas is therefore likely to interfere with the efficiency of these actions.

The PPC's primary connections are in frontal, midbrain and cerebellar areas, any of which may be affected by TBI. In turn, each of these primary connections has functional relationships with other areas of the brain that are vulnerable to damage in acceleration–deceleration injuries, such as the nuclei of the brainstem. Damage to the brainstem–cerebellar functional loop may be particularly relevant to rehabilitation practice, given the importance of these structures in recognizing the need for adaptation and in recalibrating reflexes such as the vestibulo-ocular reflex (Leigh and Zee 1991).

There is some evidence that cerebellar dysfunction may actually confound the execution of efficient movement (e.g. Day et al 1998), and we need to know much more about the effects of suboptimal function in this area on the potential for relearning and of its impact on normal experientially based automatic adaptive processes. It may be appropriate to use intact visual processes to monitor progress and action during skill acquisition, but equally the use of the same strategies in the presence of dysfunction may in fact add to errors in performance.

Knowledge of normal visual function and the recognition of visual dysfunction should be more central to our practice. Research into the impact of visual dysfunction on motor performance, along with studies analysing the effect of intervention strategies using vision, must be a priority area of attention within progressive neurophysiotherapeutic practice.

COGNITION AND BEHAVIOUR

While the nature of physiotherapy demands that we focus in on motor performance, movement is clearly only one part of human behaviour. In normal life movement is inextricably linked with functional goals and those goals are derived from a complex set of intentions, desires, needs and demands. Moreover, learning processes, including those central to the recovery of movement and skilled action after neural insult, are dependent on the function of the brain as a whole. It is important, therefore, that physiotherapists are able to take into account the influence of non-physical factors and global brain function when planning programmes to address dysfunctional motor performance.

Neuropsychology, as a profession, has attempted to develop an understanding of the relationship between brain and behaviour by systematic assessment and analysis of findings (Lezak 1995). In recent years the emergence of specialist clinical neuropsychologists has taken this process further by endeavouring to link the analysis of psychometric test results to psychosocial functioning and adaptation in real-life settings (Tupper & Cicerone 1990). Neuropsychologists are a tremendous resource for physiotherapists (Brazzelli & Della Sala 1997), as is the associated wealth of published literature which both describes the scope of cognitive and behavioural dysfunction and explores approaches to remedial or compensatory interventions.

Only one behavioural theme is introduced here by way of an example to encourage exploration of the wider literature and the development of closer working relationships between the two professions. Additional examples of the practical application of this process are described in more detail in the next chapter.

Motivation

Patient motivation is generally considered to be a key factor influencing therapeutic outcome. Indeed, lack of patient motivation is often given as a reason for lack of progress in rehabilitation and for withdrawal of treatment. Without the benefit of psychometric testing, motivation is commonly judged by behavioural observation, for example in terms of apparent disinterest in suggested activities, failure to carry out agreed tasks or overtly uncooperative behaviour within treatment sessions. However, apparent lack of motivation as assessed by behavioural presentation may be misleading, especially in the context of the common practice of attributing intent or conscious control on the part of the patient.

It is essential that therapists do not assume that the patient apparently lacking motivation has made a conscious decision not to cooperate or is pathologically unable to get going. Either of these two reasons may be valid but equally there are many other cognitive deficits and combinations of deficits that can lead to an apparently demotivated presentation. For example, the problem may lie in a variety of memory deficits, in difficulty sequencing actions, in a failure to link words with actions, or in limited awareness that a problem exists or that there is a need to do something about it.

There are differences in the ways in which each of these deficits would be addressed within a rehabilitation or adjustment programme, and limitations in many of these areas will impact on wider areas of functional activity than discrete motor performance. It is therefore important to establish as far as possible what is going on so that appropriate treatment strategies are developed, realistic goals are set and subsequent intervention has a good chance of success.

Physiotherapists are strongly encouraged to seek out a neuropsychological perspective in the presence of any suggestion of cognitive difficulty or when any behaviour imposes limitations on assessment, intervention or progress.

FUNCTIONAL ACTIVITY

Finally, in this brief review, I would like to introduce the need to consider the complex cerebral demands involved in the execution of activities of daily living and, with this in mind, to promote thought and discussion with regard to the demands we place on patients involved in rehabilitation and how we organize or coordinate demands across rehabilitation professionals.

The main questions are: what are reasonable demands to make of patients at a variety of stages in their rehabilitation programmes, and what level and mix of demands is likely to be most effective? Practically, if these questions can be answered, it should then follow that there would be more realistic goal setting and expectations of treatment outcomes.

Investigations of the interactions between motor and mental performance have begun to be reported, indicating that functional performance is dependent upon central processing and can be negatively affected by increasing cognitive demands (Andersson et al 1998). It has long been understood by physiotherapists that severely physically affected patients have difficulty combining walking and talking, but recent evidence suggests that the demands of dual tasks, be they motor or cognitive, cause significant difficulties for those with much more subtle deficits (Cicerone 1996).

The immediate effects of dual tasks and the anticipated cumulative effects of the high demands placed on those participating in a comprehensive rehabilitation programme need to be considered carefully in the design of the totality of the programme and in the evaluation of an individual's performance within the programme. However, where overall demands are high, simply reducing those demands is unlikely to be the complete answer.

Indeed, there is now some evidence of positive cognitive effects of aerobic exercise in adults after TBI (Rosenfeld 1998) and of the positive contribution of active movement in the reduction of visual and other forms of neglect (Robertson and North 1992, 1993, Robertson et al 1992, 1997). The study of all of these interactive effects is a fascinating area in which the physiotherapy profession should be deeply involved.

CONCLUSION

There is currently no comprehensive theory of motor performance upon which to build a complete evidence-based matrix of neurophysiotherapeutic intervention. There is a significant amount of existing and emerging basic scientific knowledge that may be applied to many areas of practice, at least at the level of exploratory hypotheses. Some areas of practice have attracted greater attention and this is reflected in a larger number of studies producing directly clinically applicable evidence.

There is, however, much to do to develop practice based on best evidence in neurophysiotherapy. Furthermore, as much of the published evidence is limited to studies of stroke or progressive neurological disorders, there is an even greater need for a focused programme of research and evaluation of direct relevance to TBI.

All therapists can and should contribute to this process and it is therefore essential to develop a common approach and agreed mechanisms to pool resources effectively, to facilitate communication and to document progress.

The approach proposed in this chapter is based on an open, developmental philosophy that acknowledges both experiential and experimentally derived knowledge, and which essentially anticipates cross-validation between the two traditions. A pragmatic multicomponent approach is suggested for gathering, documenting and generating evidence to enable the process and produce tangible evidence of progress.

The success of the overall project is dependent upon evidence being assessed against common standards and results being communicated in a globally digestible format. It is absolutely essential that neurophysiotherapists embrace the practice of communicating via the written word, publishing more, responding to published work in writing, and becoming comfortable with the idea of discussing uncertainties and controversial topics in the public domain.

The combination of this suggested pragmatic approach and lively, inclusive discussion should generate both clear and tentative links between scientific knowledge and specific interventions or treatment approaches. Areas requiring further investigation, and the reasons why, should be more easily identified and the relevance of new knowledge be more immediately obvious. The systematic building of evidence-based practice and reasoned enquiry in this way is tangible, manageable and has the potential for graded success, in contrast to the impossible task of looking for a complete rationale to support all aspects of practice within a partially evolved traditional conceptual approach.

Finally, having given great emphasis to science, logic and facts, it is also important to remember the following. No matter how much detail is added to the evidential base, the choice of approach for each individual circumstance and the application of a chosen technique or regime will remain a skillful art.

Effective TBI physiotherapists, therefore, not only need to understand and use the world of science to develop and test theories and the knowledge base, but also need to have the ability to make balanced judgements and to develop the advanced physical and interpersonal skills required to deliver the chosen intervention. As a contribution to the wider decision-making process, the next chapter examines some of the non-physical factors that influence the design and delivery of intervention programmes.

REFERENCES

Ada L, Canning C, Paratz J 1990 Care of the unconscious head-injured patient. In: Ada L, Canning C (eds) Key issues in neurological physiotherapy, 1st edn. Butterworth–Heinemann, London, p 249

Akeson W H, Amiel D, Woo S L-Y 1980 Immobility effects on synovial joints. Biorheology 17:95–110

Andersson G, Yardley L, Luxon L 1998 A dual-task study of interference between mental activity and control of balance. American Journal of Otology 19(5):632–637

Beevor C E 1904 The Croonian lectures. Adlard, London

Berger W, Hortsmann G, Dietz V 1984 Tension development and muscle activation in the leg during gait in spastic hemiparesis: independence of muscle hypertonia and exaggerated stretch reflexes. Journal of Neurology, Neurosurgery and Psychiatry 47:1029–1033

Bernard P, Dill H, Held J M, Judd D L M, Nalette E 1984 Reduction of hypertonicity by early casting in a comatose head injured individual: a case report. Physical Therapy 64:1540–1542

Bobath B 1978 Adult hemiplegia: evaluation and treatment. William Heinemann, London

Booth B J, Doyle M, Montgomery J 1983 Serial casting for the management of spasticity in the head injured patient. Physical Therapy 63:1960–1966

Brazzelli M, Della Sala S 1997 Physiotherapy and neuropsychology: an interaction that could ease the remedy of brain disease. Physiotherapy Theory and Practice 13:243–246

Brown P 1994 Pathophysiology of spasticity. Journal of Neurology, Neurosurgery and Psychiatry 57:773–777

Carey J R, Burghardt T P 1993 Movement dysfunction following central nervou system lesions: a problem of neurologic or muscular impairment. Physical Therapy 73:538–547

Carr J H, Shepherd R B 1987 Movement science: foundations for physical therapy in rehabilitation, 1st edn. Aspen, Rockville

Carr J H, Shepherd R B (eds) 1998 Neurological rehabilitation: optimizing motor performance, 1st edn. Butterworth–Heinemann, Oxford

Cicerone K D 1996 Attentional deficits and dual task demands after mild traumatic brain injury. Brain Injury 10(2):79–89

Citta-Pietrolungo T J, Alexander M A, Steg N L 1992 Early detection of heterotopic ossification in young patients with traumatic brain injury. Archives of Physical Medicine and Rehabilitation 73:258–262

Collin C, Daly G 1998 Brain injury. In: Stokes M (ed) Neurological physiotherapy. Mosby, London, p 91

Conine T A, Sullivan T, Mackie T, Goodman M 1990 Effect of serial casting for the prevention of equinus in patients with acute head injury. Archives of Physical Medicine and Rehabilitation 71:310–312

Cornall C 1992 Splinting and contractures. Synapse April:50–54

Day B L, Thompsom P D, Harding A E, Marsden C D 1998 Influence of vision on upperlimb reaching movements in patients with cerebellar ataxia. Brain 121:357–372

Dieber M P, Passingham R E, Colebatch J G, Friston K J, Nixon P D, Frackowiak R S J 1991 Cortical area and the selection of movement: a study with positron emission tomography. Experimental Brain Research 84:393–402

Dietz V 1995 Compensatory reflex mechanisms following limb displacements. In: Cody F W J (ed) Neural control of skilled human movement, 1st edn. Portland Press, London, p 51

Dietz V, Quintern J, Berger W 1981 Electrophysiological studies of gait in spasticity and rigidity. Evidence that altered mechanical properties of muscle contribute to hypertonia. Brain 104:431–449

Edwards S, Charlton P 1996 Splinting and the use of orthoses in the management of patients with neurological disorders. In: Edwards S (ed) Neurological physiotherapy: a problem solving approach, 1st edn. Churchill Livingstone, New York, p 161

Ellis E 1990 Respiratory function following head injury. In: Ada L, Canning C (eds) Key issues in neurological physiotherapy, 1st edn. Butterworth–Heinemann, London, p 237

Frost E A M 1985 Management of head injury. Canadian Anaesthetic Society Journal 32(3):532

Gandevia S C, Burke D 1984 Saturation in human somatosensory pathways. Experimental Brain Research 54:582

Gandevia S, McCloskey D, Burke D 1992 Kinesthetic signals and muscle contraction. Trends in Neuroscience 15(2):62–65

Garrad J, Bullock M 1986 The effect of respiratory therapy on intracranial pressure in ventilated neurosurgical patients. Australian Journal of Physiotherapy 32(2):107–111

Goldspink G, Williams P 1990 Muscle fibre changes and connective tissue changes associated with use and disuse. In: Ada L, Canning C (eds) Key issues in neurological physiotherapy, 1st edn. Butterworth–Heinemann, London, p 197

Gordon J 1990 Disorders of motor control. In: Ada L, Canning C (eds) Key issues in neurological physiotherapy, 1st edn. Butterworth–Heinemann, London, p 25

Grafton S T, Mazziotta J, Presty S, Friston K J, Frackowiak R S J, Phelps M E 1992 Functional anatomy of human procedural learning determined with regional cerebral blood flow and PET. Journal of Neuroscience 12:2542–2548

Hillier S, Sharpe M, Metzer J 1997 Outcomes 5 years post-traumatic brain injury (with further reference to neurophysical impairment and disability). Brain Injury 11(9):661–675

Hurvitz E A, Mandac B R, Davidoff G, Johnson J H, Nelson V S 1992 Risk factors for heterotropic ossification in children and adolescents with severe traumatic brain injury. Archives of Physical Medicine and Rehabilitation 73:459–462

Jueptner M, Weiller C 1998 A review of differences between basal ganglia and cerebellar control of movements as revealed by functional imaging studies. Brain 121:1437–1449

Kabat H, Knott M 1954 Proprioceptive facilitation therapy for paralysis. Physiotherapy 40:171–176

Karni A, Bertini G 1997 Learning perceptual skills: behavioural probes into adult cortical plasticity. Current Opinion in Neurobiology 7(4):530–535

Karni A, Meyer G, Jezzard P, Adams M M, Turner R, Ungerleider L G 1995 Functional MRI evidence for adult motor cortex plasticity during motor skill learning. Nature 377:155–158

Kidd G, Lawes N, Musa I (eds) Understanding neuromuscular plasticity, 1st edn. Edward Arnold, London

Kopelman M D, Stevens T G, Foli S, Grasby P 1998 PET activation of the medial temporal lobe in learning. Brain 121:875–887

Latash M L 1993 Examples of motor disorders. In: Control of human movement, 1st edn. Human Kinetics, Champaign, IL, p 263

Leigh R J, Zee D S (eds) 1991 The neurology of eye movements, 2nd edn. F A Davis, Philadelphia, PA

Lemon R N 1995 Cortical control of skilled movements. In: Cody F W J (ed) Neural control of skilled human movements, 1st edn. Portland Press, London, p 1

Lezak M D 1995 Neuropsychological assessment, 3rd edn. Oxford University Press, New York

Lunn J N 1991 Lecture notes on anaesthetics, 4th edn. Blackwell Scientific, Oxford

McLellan D L 1993 Rehabilitation in neurology. In: Walton J (ed) Brain's disorders of the nervous system, 10th edn. Oxford University Press, Oxford, p 768

Magnus R 1926 Some results of studies in the physiology of posture. Lancet ii:531–536, 585–588

Mills V 1984 Electromyographic results of inhibitory splinting. Physical Therapy 64:190–207

Moritatani T, deVries H A 1979 Neural factors versus hypertrophy in the time course of muscle strength gain. American Journal of Physical Medicine 58:115–130

Moseley A M 1997 The effect of casting combined with stretching on passive ankle dorsiflexion in adults with traumatic brain injury. Physical Therapy 77:240–247

Nadler M A, Harrison L M, Stephens J A 1998 Acquisition of a new motor skill is accompanied by changes in the cortical components of cutaneomuscular reflexes from finger muscles in man. University of East London, London

O'Dwyer N J, Ada L, Neilson P D 1996 Spasticity and muscle contracture following stroke. Brain 119(5):1737–1749

Paratz J, Burns Y 1993 The effect of respiratory physiotherapy on intracranial pressure, mean arterial pressure, cerebral perfusion pressure and end tidal carbon dioxide in ventilated neurosurgical patients. Physiotherapy Theory and Practice 9:3–11

Partridge C J 1996 Physiotherapy approaches to the treatment of neurological conditions – an historical perspective. In: Edwards S (ed) Neurological physiotherapy: a problem solving approach, 1st edn. Churchill Livingstone, New York, p 3

Passingham R E 1987 Motor areas of the cerebral cortex. John Wiley, Chichester, UK

Pette D, Vrbova G 1985 Neural control of phenotype expression in mammalian muscle fibres. Muscle Nerve 8:676–689

Plant R 1998 Theoretical basis of treatment concepts. In: Stokes M (ed) Neurological physiotherapy, 1st edn. Mosby, London, p 271

Pope P 1992 Management of the physical condition in patients with chronic and severe neurological pathologies. Physiotherapy 78(12):896–903

Robertson I H, North N 1992 Spatio-motor cueing in unilateral left neglect: the role of hemispace, hand and motor activation. Neuropsychologia 30(6):553–563

Robertson I H, North N 1993 Active and passive activation of left limbs: influence on visual and sensory neglect. Neuropsychologia 31(3):293–300

Robertson I H, North N T, Geggie C 1992 Spatiomotor cueing in unilateral left neglect: three case studies of its therapeutic effects. Journal of Neurology, Neurosurgery and Psychiatry 55(9):799–805

Robertson I H, Nico D, Hood B M 1997 Believing what you feel: using proprioceptive feedback to reduce unilateral neglect. Neuropsychology 11(1):53–58

Rood M S 1954 Neurophysiologic reactions: a basis for physical therapy. Physical Therapy Review 34:444–449

Rosenfeld J 1998 Psychological/cognitive benefits of aerobic training. University of East London, London

Rusk H A, Loman E W, Block J M 1966 Rehabilitation of the patient with head injury. Clinical Neurosurgery 12:312–323

Schluter N D, Rushworth M F S, Passingham R E, Mills K R 1998 Temporary interference in human lateral premotor cortex suggests dominance for the selection of movements: a study using transcranial magnetic stimulation. Brain 121:785–799

Sherrington C S 1913 Reflex inhibition as a factor in the co-ordination of movements and postures. Quarterly Journal of Experimental Physiology 6:251

Sherrington C S 1947 The integrative action of the nervous system. Cambridge University Press, Cambridge

Shumway-Cook A, Woollacott M (eds) 1995 Motor control – theory and practical applications. Williams & Wilkins, Baltimore, MD

Stein J F 1992 The representation of egocentric space in the posterior parietal cortex. Behavioural Brain Sciences 15:691–700

Stein J 1995 The posterior parietal cortex, the cerebellum and the visual guidance of movement. In: Cody F W J (ed) Neural control of skilled human movement, 1st edn. Portland Press, Chichester, UK, p 31

Sullivan T, Conine T A, Goodman M, Mackie T 1988 Serial casting to prevent equinus in acute traumatic head injury. Physiotherapy Canada 40:346–350

Thilman A F, Fellows S J, Ross H F 1991 Biomechanical changes at the ankle joint after stroke. Journal of Neurology, Neurosurgery and Psychiatry 54:134–139

Tupper D E, Cicerone K D (eds) 1990 The neuropsychology of everyday life, 1st edn. Kluwer Academic Publishers, Boston, MA

Vrbova G, Gordon T, Jones R 1978 Nerve–muscle interaction. Chapman & Hall, London

Wood R L 1991 Critical analysis of the concept of sensory stimulation for patients in vegetative states. Brain Injury 5(4):401–409

Cognitive, behavioural and individual influences in programme design

Key Points

- The presence of cognitive limitations places additional professional responsibilities on physiotherapists in terms of consent to treatment and in the conduct of therapeutic interactions
- The potential impact of cognitive or behavioural dysfunction should be considered in advance of any therapeutic interaction, and relevant management strategies should be identified and executed as appropriate
- Decisions concerning therapeutic goals and the design and content of individual sessions should take due account of current cognitive and behavioural issues
- Physiotherapy interventions can be valuable in facilitating or achieving non-physical goals

INTRODUCTION

The influence of cognitive limitations or behavioural difficulties, which are experienced by many people who sustain a traumatic brain injury (TBI), must be taken into account during the assessment for, and the design and delivery of, a planned physical programme.

The impact of difficulties within the cognitive–behavioural spectrum may be felt at any point in the therapeutic process. It is therefore pertinent to anticipate what that impact may be even before any direct contact is established and to make preparations to help ensure the successful conduct of the assessment, a relevant approach within direct therapeutic sessions and suitable content and design for a home programme. This type of groundwork is also essential to inform evaluation of progress and judgement of success and will prove valuable even for discharge planning and the organization of any postdischarge review.

For each facet of therapeutic practice, from assessment to long-term management, there is potentially a complex range of deficit profiles, raising many different issues and requiring a variety of responses. Since this precludes comprehensive coverage within a single chapter, what is presented here is an overview of some of the issues for physiotherapists raised by the presence of cognitive dysfunction in each of the stages of contact, together with discussion of some of the common behavioural manifestations of underlying cognitive deficits.

Management strategies helpful in achieving physical goals are described and there is also discussion of how physical interventions may be used to facilitate other types of team goals. There is little published work linking cognitive function and physical intervention, so I have opted to present suggestions based on clinical experience of addressing the complex interaction of deficits seen in many individuals participating in rehabilitation and adjustment programmes.

As before, case examples are used to highlight specific issues and to illustrate a cohesive approach to a complete set of strengths and limitations as identified by the interdisciplinary assessment. Although particular elements of dysfunction and/or behavioural presentation are highlighted in separate sections, it should be appreciated that many of the issues have an impact at virtually all stages of the process.

ANTICIPATING FACTORS THAT WILL AFFECT THE THERAPEUTIC INTERACTION

Cognitive dysfunction may impact on the therapeutic relationship before the initial meeting between therapist and client. In Chapter 3 we discussed the skewed control relationship between professionals and service users in emergency care created by the need for speedy, informed, decision making with regard to medical intervention and often, in the case of more severe injuries, complicated by the patient's altered state of consciousness. Working with a person whose conscious level remains depressed, or who has cognitive limitations, places added responsibility on the therapist in terms of consent to treatment and in the conduct of interactions.

CONSENT TO TREATMENT

Increasingly, documented guidance governing consent to treatment and interactions between healthcare professionals and vulnerable adults, such as those with cognitive dysfunction following TBI, is being produced within individual organizations. However, even where guidelines are available, they are likely to contain phrases such as *professional judgement* or *standard care*, which are open to interpretation, especially where there is a paucity of published literature. Therapists must make themselves aware of the legal and professional issues around informed consent, press for the development of local guidelines and ensure that their practice is defensible.

Where there is practice innovation or possible controversy regarding treatment choice, it is advisable to document the decision-making process and to record the agreement of a comparable or more senior practitioner. These cautions apply where the injured person remains deeply unconscious, for example when applying casts or splints, and also at times of fluctuating consciousness or when there is any level of confusion.

This approach may appear cumbersome and a formal process may not be deemed necessary when there is confidence that interventions are of a standard nature and would be judged as such by a group of peers. However, the principle is that when the injured person is not in the position to agree or refuse treatment from an informed standpoint there must be another mechanism to help ensure they receive best care and to offer protection to them and to healthcare practitioners alike. Such a mechanism should be based on standards of professional conduct, available practice guidelines and clear, appropriately detailed, clinical notes.

CONDUCT OF THERAPEUTIC INTERACTIONS

In the same way that it is necessary, in the presence of cognitive dysfunction, to give additional thought to the process of consent to treatment, physiotherapists must also be aware of the impact of their own behaviour on the progress and outcome of any therapeutic interaction. Therapists' ability to modify their approach to intervention and their behaviour within treatment sessions appropriate to the needs of the injured person will have an impact in terms of the immediate tolerance of treatment and subsequently in terms of positive outcome. Conversely, any failure to achieve an adequate balance within a therapeutic interaction or to choose or apply an approach appropriate to the particular requirements of an individual case may have a lasting negative effect (see Case example 9.1).

POSITIVE PREPARATION

The success of any therapeutic interaction can be affected positively by anticipating the factors that may influence the injured person's initial presentation or behaviour during the interaction. This is important to consider throughout the period of contact, but it is arguably of particular importance in establishing the level of communication required to begin to develop a therapeutic alliance at the earliest opportunity.

Consideration should be given to what type of cognitive–behavioural factors may be encountered and what strategies might be brought to bear to manage them positively. Adequate preparation will help ensure a good outcome in terms of both parties feeling positive about current and future sessions and the achievement of objectives set for the current session.

Preparation for an initial subacute session

In subacute provision, therapists have what might be loosely termed a captive audience: the injured person is resident onsite. Theoretically, this offers the opportunity for a variety of different approaches to developing a working relationship, for example by spending a lengthy initial period gathering assessment information slowly or by opting for multiple short visits over the working day.

The decision of what constitutes an appropriate approach for an individual case and what might be reasonable objectives to set for each contact session should be based on the type of preassessment information gathering described in the earlier chapters of this book. Thus, the reported observations of medical, nursing and other colleagues within the wider rehabilitation team should directly inform the physiotherapist's initial plan of contact. An example of this process is given in Table 9.1.

Preparation for an initial post-acute session

The non-residential status of clients referred for assessment to any outpatient programme offers a particular challenge as this client group has a reputation for erratic or non-attendance. Therefore, when the person to be assessed is living in the wider community, precontact preparations, in addition to planning the content and execution of the contact session, must include consideration of how best to ensure that attendance for assessment is achieved.

In individual cases, referral sources may provide specific information outlining cognitive difficulties, behavioural traits or family issues that may act as potential barriers to attendance. This type of information can be used to tailor the initial communication process appropriately, for example confirming the first appointment via a social worker or other professional already known to the client or family.

Table 9.1 Example of planning the initial approach in subacute care

Available information	Influence on approach	Initial plan
Patient is: Disoriented in place and time	Aim: Not to increase the levels of confusion or agitation	First establish contact in the most familiar environment (i.e. do not remove to therapy department)
Sometimes agitated Sometimes able to engage in social conversation	To use preserved conversational skills	Give a simple explanation of who you are and what your role is (repeat as necessary)
		Do not proceed to physical examination if agitation is significant or increasing
		Be prepared to have a high ratio of reassurance time in comparison to active physical assessment
		Be prepared to gather information over multiple contacts
		Observe spontaneous motor performance and any factors associated with increasing confusion or agitation
		Leave some record of the visit (e.g. a note of your name and when you will return or a photograph saying who and what you are)

However, even without specific guidance, given knowledge of the pathophysiology of TBI and the almost universal prevalence of dysfunction in memory skills and organizational abilities, for example, it is reasonable to anticipate that anyone who has had a significant TBI may experience practical difficulties in responding appropriately to an appointment letter. It is useful, therefore, to build safeguards into the process of allocating and confirming appointments and in getting clients to the first, and often subsequent, appointment.

An example of how memory dysfunction can affect compliance in attending the first outpatient appointment and some compensatory strategies that can be used to control for these difficulties are given in Table 9.2.

Dealing with established issues

Previous experience can have a strong impact on subsequent attitudes. Therefore, where it is known, for example, that the injured person or their family had a negative experience of health services before their contact with your service, it is useful to take specific action to deal with the effects of their negative experience. This may involve early discussion of the

Table 9.2   Impact of memory dysfunction on outpatient attendance

Primary problem	Manifestation	Compensatory strategies
Memory dysfunction	Reads the appointment letter and then completely forgets having received it	Ask for a family member or friend to attend the first appointment
		Include a prepaid reply card with appointment letter to confirm attendance and make telephone contact if reply not forthcoming; then
		Offer to telephone on the morning of the appointment to prompt recall
		If providing transport, encourage transport driver to make contact with your service before leaving the client's home if there is confusion about attendance
	Fails to remember it is the day for the appointment	Ensure appointment details also go to a family member or friend
		Include an offer of transport to the first appointment
		Make the appointment for morning so that the transport arrives before the client leaves the house to do something else

problem with appropriate reassurance or, in some cases, an overt demonstration of a different approach that will, without the need for discussion, relieve anxiety.

In the same way, where there is a known behavioural problem, say, involving frequent visits to the toilet or frequent requests for coffee or cigarettes, it is useful to devise in advance an initial strategy to deal with these predictable requests.

This may involve an attempt to get agreement on a reasonable frequency of breaks or the decision to make a clear statement about what constitutes the normal session length and how often breaks are timetabled. Alternatively it may be decided that it is important to establish a behavioural baseline, which would involve simply documenting the frequency of requests without any attempt to influence the behaviour. If the latter is the case then the physical objectives of the session may have to be regarded as secondary, thus altering the expectations of what constitutes a successful outcome for the session.

The important thing is to decide on the approach in advance and to make every effort to put the agreed approach into practice. Failure to prepare or to adopt a consistent approach will only lead to confusion for therapist and client alike.

FACTORS INFLUENCING THE CONDUCT AND OUTCOME OF THE PHYSICAL ASSESSMENT

Some of the special considerations that apply to assessment design and content have been discussed in earlier chapters. What is presented here is concerned more with the direct interaction between the physiotherapist and the injured person during assessment sessions and, in particular, how cognitive deficits can influence behavioural presentation. We will also briefly discuss the need for a skilled response to some of the behaviours described and a related need for caution in the interpretation of some of these and other observed behaviours.

MOOD, BEHAVIOUR AND COGNITION

Perhaps one of the most difficult aspects of behavioural presentation for physically based therapists to understand, and to allow for, is the concept that behaviour may reflect an underlying reflex, autonomic or cognitive process rather than a reasoned intention to act. Although the whole question of how much human beings are in control of behaviour – what proportion of actions is dictated by reflex, chemical or other preprogrammed responses and what proportion involves choice or volition – has been a focus for philosophers and academics throughout history, much still remains unanswered.

However, it is clear that normal adult human behaviour comprises simple reflex and more complex automatic behaviours as well as those that are consciously volitional. What is also clear is that any single factor or set of factors that changes the capacity for the brain to work in a normal way can result in perceptual and/or behavioural change. For example, the ingestion of alcohol or various drugs, chemical inhalation, sleep deprivation or fever can all produce changes in behaviour or cognition ranging from relatively minor changes in behavioural presentation through obvious changes in perceptuomotor skills, erratic or irrational behaviours, to coma, and death.

All of these cognitive–behavioural changes reflect either subtle or more substantial disruption of normal brain function, and while the provoking conditions remain active much of the resultant behaviour is beyond conscious and/or reasoned volitional control.

In the same way, TBI provokes structural and biochemical changes that can lead to temporary and/or permanent changes in brain function. Deficits resulting from each area of malfunctioning brain may be identified via systematic evaluation of complex skills or their component parts (as in formal assessment) but equally the combined effect of the underlying deficits may be observed in behaviour and/or functional performance.

It follows, therefore, that observed abnormal or changed behaviours, like disordered physical function, may have their basis in cerebral dysfunction. It also follows that some behaviours, like some physical skills, are barely under control and remain vulnerable to environmental change. Furthermore, other behaviours, like some physical activities, may not yet be mastered and the ability to use them appropriately in everyday life may continue to prove elusive.

It is essential, then, that physiotherapists consider the contribution of underlying cognitive dysfunction in the production of negative or disruptive behaviours as this can often offer both explanation and potential management solutions. Some examples of behavioural presentations and possible underlying cognitive deficits are given in Table 9.3.

WORKING WITH COGNITIVE AND BEHAVIOURAL DYSFUNCTION

Being aware of the impact of cognitive and behavioural dysfunction allows the physiotherapist to control for these factors within the process of assessment and to interpret how the injured person presents from a wider perspective. The examples given in the preceding section, connected with

Table 9.3   Behavioural presentations and some possible underlying cognitive limitations

Behaviour or presentation	Associated cognitive limitations
Agitated behaviour (physical or verbal)	Still in post-traumatic amnesia Confusion as a result of perceptual difficulties Confusion as a result of memory difficulties Heightened state of arousal (upset, angry, worried) with difficulty returning to a calmer state without external assistance Unable to sustain attention
Boredom or disinterest	Still in post-traumatic amnesia Low state of arousal Difficulty initiating activity Problems with non-verbal communication Unable to sustain attention Slow information processing
Repetitive speech	Perseveration Memory problems Anxiety
Quiet, not forthcoming in discussion	Word-finding difficulties Memory problems Orientation problems Fatigue

advance preparation, are illustrative of methods of control that seek either to reduce the immediate demand on the individual, or to offer increased levels of support to them. The primary principle underpinning these strategies and most of the methods suggested throughout the rest of this chapter involve the manipulation of the environment external to the injured person to facilitate a positive outcome in terms of either their immediate participation or improved function.

Applying this principle to the conduct of the face-to-face assessment session largely entails the physiotherapist skilfully conducting the session in a flexible manner. This may include adjustments of pace, simplification of language, the use of gesture and demonstration, or other modifications of personal behaviour. Often, experienced therapists do all of these things, almost as second nature, while others may fail to make any or all of the necessary adjustments, leading to lack of success, frustration and possibly an escalation of negative behaviours (see Case example 9.1).

The counterproductive nature of the therapist not getting the conduct of the interaction quite right is patently clear but there is also potential danger when an intuitive practitioner fails to acknowledge the adjustment and behavioural modifications that they make. This lack of awareness may lead to an overestimation of the level at which the injured person is performing and this in turn can result in the production of an over-demanding programme.

There are many other implications of failing to appreciate the extent of someone's cognitive limitations, including reaching inaccurate conclusions about levels of motivation, interest and commitment, the unnecessary provocation of behavioural outbursts, and inadequate preparation for new activities or placements. One very significant outcome of professionals failing to appreciate the extent of an injured person's cognitive difficulties is the underestimation of the effort and energy required of family members in having constantly to make adjustments to support optimum function or prevent behavioural difficulties.

Some examples of cognitive dysfunction and appropriate adjustment strategies to help ensure a successful conclusion to an assessment session are given in Table 9.4.

The problem of professionals underestimating difficulties is not confined to cases where the injured person is mobile and apparently operating at a relatively high level, masking underlying problems. Case example 9.1, as well as placing some of the already highlighted issues in context, also illustrates a failure to appreciate that the demands being placed on a severely injured young man were not entirely appropriate and were contributing to difficulties in management. Some of the resultant negative effects are described along with evidence to support the possibility of reversing negative behaviours, even in the presence of severe damage and at a substantial time after injury.

Table 9.4 Adjusting to compensate for cognitive limitations

Cognitive limitation or issue	Therapist's adjustments or strategies
Diminished speed and capacity for information processing	Slow the pace of speech, do not use complex sentences Allow extra time for response, tolerate silence Do not ask supplementary questions before receiving the initial response Monitor for signs of tiring Punctuate the session with short breaks
Lengthy period of post-traumatic amnesia	Establish when day-to-day recall returned; do not pursue questions about progress during the period of post-traumatic amnesia; do not record as fact the injured person's report of events during the period of amnesia Give reassurance that lack of, or patchy, recall during this period is to be expected Where possible, obtain factual information from other sources about significant events during the period of limited recall to aid discussions of progress
Ongoing memory dysfunction	Do not rely solely on free self-report of difficulties Test or obtain corroboration of true functional level Repeat explanations and other reassuring information as necessary Use written materials
Language comprehension problems	Use simple language, relevant to the immediate context Add gesture and physical demonstration or by way of video recordings Use diagrams
Attentional problems	Work for short periods with rests Modify the environment to minimize intrusions and distractions (noise, other activities within the field of vision, unplanned interruptions) Use specific cues to promote attention (tactile, visual, auditory, active movement)

Case example 9.1   Craig

As part of the planning of a long-term management programme, I was asked to provide an independent opinion on Craig's physical status and physiotherapeutic needs. He had sustained a very serious injury almost 6 years previously at the age of 17, and had only recently moved home into newly purchased single-level accommodation. When I saw Craig he was essentially bed–chair-bound. He communicated via gesture and some vocalizations, but had no clear words and, at that time, no communication aids. Before the assessment I was warned that he could be behaviourally difficult.

When I first arrived in Craig's house he was being assisted, by a carer who was well known to him, to take a drink. He was in a modified long sitting position on top of his bed. I was introduced to Craig by his carer and it was explained that I had come to make an assessment. Craig took my hand and made a good attempt at kissing the back of it. It was established that I was welcome to sit in on the interaction that was underway and I was able to observe how Craig and his carer communicated as well as to note spontaneous movements and postural habits.

> **Case example 9.1** *Cont'd*
>
> During the interaction between Craig and his carer, movement was observed as occurring only in the right limbs and, throughout the whole of their period of contact, Craig looked only to the right where his carer was sitting or held his head central and flexed slightly forward. Clinical notes also described Craig as consistently failing to attend to the left side of his environment.
>
> Before beginning my assessment I began to explain what I was about to do, and at this point I was standing in a similar position to where Craig's carer had previously been. He again took hold of my hand and appeared to be interested in what I had to say. However, within my explanation I used the word physiotherapist and immediately Craig's muscle tone elevated, he closed his eyes and turned his head away towards the left and firmly held this position, refusing to re-establish any direct contact with me.
>
> It was only after substantial negotiation with Craig's mother and his carers that he eventually reluctantly agreed to a brief physical examination. Although he cooperated in a passive way, he continued to refuse to communicate directly with me.

Discussion of Case example 9.1

A review of Craig's postinjury progress and rehabilitation history revealed that he had been consecutively placed in three inpatient facilities since the time of his injury. He was in acute care for most of the first year, a hospital rehabilitation ward for 4 months and then an independent community-based care and rehabilitation facility for 4 years. He had remained deeply unconscious for many months, and that had been followed by several months of apparent fluctuating awareness of his environment. However, while in the hospital rehabilitation ward he was tolerating supported standing for substantial periods in the day and this continued in the early period in the community-based facility.

Craig became increasingly aware of his environment over the early period in the community and occasional difficult behaviours were documented, but they were not sustained and did not disrupt his ongoing programme. The behaviours were referred to in a report of a medical review, along with the rehabilitation consultant's opinion that they were probably manifestations of his reasonable distress as a result of his increasing awareness of his situation. In the same report Craig was also documented as using reliable hand signals to indicate yes or no.

A number of things then occurred that, in retrospect, could be seen to coincide with escalating behavioural difficulties and with subsequent regression in physical and communicative performance. There was a change in therapy staff, first in speech therapy and then in physiotherapy.

The new speech therapist tried to introduce the use of an electronic speech aid, which was eventually abandoned after several months, being judged as too difficult for Craig to manage. Craig started to refuse to attend physiotherapy and would hit out and attempt to bite the new physiotherapist.

Eventually he would begin to make noise and demonstrate physical agitation when her voice could be heard outside his room. Initially, the response was to force Craig to go to the treatment area until, following a period of substantial conflict, he was left to his own devices.

Craig's family and carers' assessment of the situation was that the new physiotherapist did not engage with Craig as an individual, did not allow him the time he needed to respond to requests or direction, and interpreted his slowness as him not being cooperative. She spent increasingly less time directly with him, leaving assistant staff to carry out repetitive activities (which had no obvious functional purpose). The family's opinion was that Craig was frustrated, that he felt rejected and ignored, and that he was bored.

It is, of course, not possible to determine with absolute certainty what exactly caused Craig's negative behaviours to escalate, but it is clear that both the new therapists failed to establish a constructive therapeutic relationship with Craig and that physiotherapy (as well as attempts to use the electronic communicator) became synonymous with negative experience. Eventually independent expert advice on behavioural management was sought but Craig's behaviours were by this time rigidly established and assessed as being so firmly linked with the whole environment that the cycle could be broken only by removing him from that environment.

Both the development of problem behaviours and the difficulties in breaking the negative cycle were strongly influenced by Craig's cognitive limitations and communicative difficulties. For example, the failure to establish effective communication helped promote Craig's need to use protest behaviour, and his processing and language difficulties severely restricted the possibilities for reasoned discussion.

Craig was working at a very concrete level, understanding only what he actually experienced and not being able to see the long-term consequences of his actions. He was thought to be at least partially aware of his changed circumstances (recalling preinjury people and events) and to be, at times, distressed as a result. He was being repeatedly presented with the task of using a communication aid that proved to be too complex for him, and the two therapists that he had been working well with on an almost daily basis over many months had disappeared from his life in quick succession.

It is possible that the behaviours presented to the new physiotherapist initially had their basis in the wider issues that Craig was trying to deal with. However, in this case the behaviours were seen primarily as a refusal of physiotherapy treatment and, as the daily regime was regarded as an essential part of his management, attempts were made to override his apparent refusal, causing the development of a conflict relationship between Craig and his physiotherapist. Craig's avoidance behaviours were obvious, but equally the therapist's behaviour of devolving the majority of direct contact to other staff is suggestive that she may have found their interactions just as unsatisfactory.

There was no overall analysis (by the treating team) of possible provoking factors for the escalating behavioural difficulties and it was not until the whole therapeutic situation had broken down that advice was sought, by which time Craig's negative behaviours were numerous and occurred in many situations.

It is positive to record that, following the change in Craig's living environment and the re-establishment of basic communication at a yes/no level, his protest behaviours reduced significantly. Within a settled care regime, a structured programme of physiotherapy has been slowly reintroduced, overseen by a skilled case manager. Craig is once again having a planned programme of intervention in an effort at least to regain the best level of physical status, achieved at about 2 years postinjury. In the longer term the same steady approach will be used to look again at Craig's potential to achieve a higher level of communicative expression.

CONTROLLING FOR COGNITIVE LIMITATIONS IN THE DELIVERY OF A PHYSICAL PROGRAMME

In standard practice, the physiotherapy programme is commonly designed to address physical goals and, in line with the approach promoted within this book, those goals would be derived from an inclusive assessment taking into account a variety of influencing factors. However, physiotherapeutic practice within an interdisciplinary team may well include a direct contribution to the realization of rehabilitation goals other than the purely physical.

We will consider both these aspects of physiotherapeutic practice within this brief review of the management of cognitive limitations within programme design. Therefore, in addition to discussing strategies for use within sessions focused on purely physical goals, we will also look at some examples of how physically based programmes, or the manner in which they are conducted, can be used to assist progress in achieving non-physical rehabilitation goals.

SETTING SESSION OBJECTIVES AND PLANNING INTERVENTION

We have already discussed the need to vary the content and style of the therapist's presentation in order to ensure the optimum outcome with regard to assessment. A similarly thoughtful approach remains applicable throughout the period of contact but, as there may be a significant difference between the objectives underpinning assessment and those of an active rehabilitation programme, this difference needs to be reflected in the chosen approach.

Specifically, while assessment objectives are likely to be concerned primarily with information gathering, the common goal of the majority of active rehabilitation programmes is the desire to effect change. This may mean, for example, planning to reduce the level of accommodation or support offered by therapists so that the injured person progressively takes more responsibility in ensuring the success of interactions, rather than the approach of controlling the environment to minimize unnecessary demands suggested for use during assessment.

With information and guidance provided by other members of the team, physiotherapists can contribute to social skills, behavioural management and functional communication programmes, and can learn to support a variety of strategies and management systems designed to promote optimal functional performance in the face of cognitive restrictions. Moreover, since the regular and sometimes intense periods of contact between a physiotherapist and the person recovering from a TBI may constitute a significant proportion of that person's social contact, they may have few other opportunities to put into practice new skills being learned with other team members.

The need for cross-session reinforcement and opportunities for functional application of relearned, new or vulnerable skills is, of course, equally applicable to motor skills, illustrating the interdependent nature of rehabilitation and the need for effective interdisciplinary working to achieve anything like true recovery potential. This reciprocal relationship allows skills practice in a variety of real functional situations during the course of other aspects of the programme. However, it is important to note that practice will be set at the correct level only when goals and progress are shared continuously across professionals. This again highlights the need for effective communication and for a sense of shared responsibility for the outcome of the programme as a whole.

Spending at least part of any session with this wider focus can also address, in a limited way, the issue of dual tasking, for example maintaining appropriate trunk and shoulder girdle position and optimum grip strength while planning and recording the following week's diary, or maintaining reasonable speed and rhythm of gait while discussing shopping purchases in the supermarket.

RAISING AWARENESS

Encouragement and reinforcement of non-physical goals within the physical programme can be particularly influential in cases where the achievement of physical goals is the individual's primary motivation, and especially where there is limited awareness of the value of addressing cognitive limitations. Physiotherapists often have the luxury of having very practical and tangible tasks to base their programme around and which are easily seen to be relevant by the client.

In contrast, work on more abstract cognitive issues may initially appear to the client to be irrelevant and it may be difficult for other team members to gain acceptance of either the need for, or the practical application of, a suggested programme of intervention. In these circumstances it may be possible to assist the development of the client's understanding within the delivery of the physical programme. For example, structuring the physical programme in a way that illustrates the need for improved performance concerning a vulnerable skill (such as recall of information), or the usefulness of having a compensatory technique (such as an effective recording system), can raise their awareness of the functional impact of the problem. This in turn can lead to a greater understanding of the importance of addressing the problem and, therefore, of the relevance of the intervention being offered by another team member.

This approach, along with some of the associated benefits for the progression of the physical programme, can be illustrated in practice by revisiting the case of Bryan (Case example 9.2).

Case example 9.2   Bryan

The components of the initial programme recommended for Bryan (see Case example 7.2) were to:

1. Develop a physical programme (needed and seen as valid by Bryan)
2. Establish strategies for recording activities and then for memory support (needed but not recognized by Bryan)
3. Provide education about TBI and its resultant effects.

Discussion of Case example 9.2

Establishing the physical programme

The physical programme, as well as addressing sensorimotor dysfunction, was aimed at improving mood and self-image by replicating activities of the type Bryan associated with his preinjury self. He was keen to exercise as this had always been the way in which he had made himself feel healthy, and he had also used demanding physical activities as a release for stress.

Direct intervention to ameliorate Bryan's negative symptoms and decisions on treatment progression were, of course, dependent on obtaining a clear picture of the pattern and provoking factors for his shoulder pain, headache and dizziness, and their response to intervention. Unfortunately, it quickly became obvious that Bryan's self-report was extremely unreliable as his account of problems and progress between consecutive sessions was wildly inconsistent, with no recognition on his part of this being the case.

He would, for example, report having had a headache at a time when he had been actively involved in a treatment session showing no signs of distress and conversely relate having had no problems when there was reliable evidence to the contrary. He was always keen and cooperative within sessions but showed only vague recognition of activities that were repeated from session to session. He also tended to revisit the same questions regarding how he should progress his exercise activity and when he could get back to working out at the gym.

Establishing the cognitive programme

Similar difficulty in establishing a progressive working programme was being experienced by the occupational therapist addressing the second of the three initial programme objectives. Bryan did not object to attending sessions with the occupational therapist aimed at establishing a functional recording system, although he saw his cognitive difficulties as being limited to difficulty in remembering names and recognizing faces. However, although he was compliant in attending sessions and appeared open to guidance and willing to try using a recording system, he did not manage to return with any written material from home, no matter how simple the set task. Moreover, he appeared to have little recall of being set the task in the first place.

It was, however, of note that, while he did not remember either to refer to his written prompts or reliably to bring his notebook to sessions, he did consistently bring a pair of shorts with him whenever he attended the rehabilitation centre, whether or not he had a physiotherapy session booked.

Barriers to programme development

Both active elements of the rehabilitation programme were being blocked by the functional impact of Bryan's cognitive limitations, the physical element being able to move only slowly and address limited issues and the cognitive element being at a standstill. The primary problematic issues for the physical programme were:

- A lack of reliable information necessary for the safe and efficient progression of the programme
- Time being lost within physical sessions because of questioning about important but repeatedly presented issues
- The inability to ensure avoidance of factors provoking increased symptoms or to establish any exercise habit or positive management at home.

The basic difficulty for the cognitive programme was that it was impossible to promote attention to the issues to be addressed except when in the therapy session, resulting in each session starting again at the beginning. While this lack of attention outside direct sessions also essentially applied to the physical programme, the physical sessions at least started with Bryan understanding the benefit of exercise and possessing some internal drive to take part. However, even though a degree of progress could be made within sessions and some of that progress was carried over into the following session, the cause of subsequent regressions could not be identified reliably because of his poor and inaccurate recall.

Controlling the effect of blocking issues

For the physical programme to progress, there was a clear need to establish effective communication between home and rehabilitation centre and for the method of communication not to rely on verbal reporting. This was in fact a practical example of the problems identified by the initial assessment and a reiteration of the need to achieve the second of the two initial programme objectives, which to date had met with little success.

The difference now was that we had identified both a reason and a mechanism around which to build the development of the cognitive programme. The reasoning could be explained to Bryan in relation to a set of real issues of immediate importance to him, i.e. relief of pain and improving physical ability and fitness. The mechanism could be built on his established habit of always bringing shorts when coming to the rehabilitation centre.

The benefits for both parts of the programme and for Bryan's functional outcome were clear. We had something concrete on which to base development of the cognitive programme and in the process of doing so we could hope to gather accurate information about the frequency and influencing factors concerning Bryan's debilitating symptoms and so confidently progress the physical programme. In addition, success in achieving two-way communication and in establishing a system to provide successful prompts for activity at home would allow longer-term treatment planning to include the confident use of home and community-based activities as appropriate to the needs of the programme goals.

Implementing the composite programme

The need for the recording system was explained to Bryan, highlighting the following components as necessary for the success of the physical programme:

- Records of pain or dizziness, noting the current or previous activity, to be recorded as they occurred and brought to the next session
- A system for keeping written details of home exercise so he would be clear about what he had to do
- A system for reviewing and updating home exercise
- A system for writing down questions to ask therapists at the time they occurred to him

- A system to help him remember to bring, and to ask, the written questions or to present any other information that needed to be passed on
- A system for recording summary answers to important questions so that they could be read when the same thought occurred again (and he may have forgotten the answer).

The overall need was described briefly within a treatment session with both therapists in attendance and the link frequently reinforced within subsequent individual sessions. Each of the elements was introduced over a period of time, being ordered relevant to the immediate needs of the physical programme.

With Bryan's permission, a similar detailed explanation of the reasoning and the plan of action was discussed with his partner, first in theory and then over several home visits as each of the pieces was put in place. New strategies were introduced by the occupational therapist and these were quickly followed by a practical trial related to the physical programme.

The initial work was focused around a small notebook/diary, which was housed at home on a bedside table, packed with the shorts to come to the centre and reviewed by each therapist at the beginning of each session. This developed into a slightly larger folder, capable of housing A5-sized exercise sheets, with additional sections for messages, items for action and eventually a weekly planner.

Initially, physical sessions were split between direct intervention to manage the pain issues and repetitive practice of a very limited home programme based around achieving (active) postural alignment. Progress in physical terms was initially slow, with the primary aim of achieving a reliable frequency and accuracy of practice, and this took 2–3 months. During this early stage Bryan would attend the centre on 2 or 3 days each week and he would also have a home visit from one of the therapists, with his partner in attendance.

With the *process* established, the system supported Bryan through a shoulder–neck programme, a programme using eye movements and habituation activities to decrease the frequency and intensity of dizziness, and eventually a programme to improve overall conditioning, coordination and community mobility. By the time of discharge, the system had again been refined into two folders which remained at home, one for exercise sheets and one for other reference material and a small diary, which he always carried and used for appointments, specific prompts and brief notes.

Retrospective analysis

Bryan's initial symptoms were difficult to pin down and were interrelated biomechanically and behaviourally. The recording allowed us to identify patterns of occurrence and links between symptoms, and, importantly, to illustrate those links and some of the provoking factors to Bryan. The understanding that developed from this ensured a high level of compliance with the suggested programme and, with the aid of the fully developed planning and prompting system, he was able to put his intentions into practice.

The contribution to his own therapy made by Bryan at home made it possible to tackle each of his physical difficulties with a maximum of three physiotherapy contacts per week early in the programme, quickly reducing in frequency thereafter. Contact levels fluctuated over almost a 2-year period of contact. With an established exercise habit and him understanding his role in managing his residual difficulties, he was, at times when the demands of the wider programme did not allow a primary focus on physical issues, able to maintain his optimum physical status with only background physiotherapeutic support.

However, he did run into problems when dealing with unexpected events and at times when he was not able to maintain his preferred routine, for example when trying to get back on track after some days in bed with flu or in dealing with a sudden increase in headache and shoulder symptoms during a holiday when he had opted to have a break from his maintenance programme.

Bryan progressed significantly throughout the period of his rehabilitation programme but it was clear at the time of discharge that, to maintain his perceived level of independence and for him to continue to be able to participate in decision making regarding his daily life, he needed to maintain a highly structured existence. It was also clear that while he was established in his routine he needed little external assistance but that he could not effectively re-establish a routine if for any reason it was interrupted.

Bryan's case highlights the type of low-level ad hoc maintenance required over a lifetime that is suggested in Chapter 10.

MANAGING THE DAILY INFLUENCE OF COGNITIVE LIMITATIONS

So far in this chapter we have examined the influence of cognitive and behavioural issues as they relate to specific types of therapeutic interaction such as assessment, and we have illustrated some of the links between cognitive dysfunction and behavioural presentation. We have described some examples of planning strategies and collaborative programme development both to address deficits and to help control their negative impact on the overall progress of a physical programme. As a final discussion focus in this chapter, we will discuss the use of management strategies for regular use in and around direct therapy sessions.

As previously described, most of the proposed management strategies involve some manipulation of the environment external to the injured person. In this context the external environment comprises both the physical surroundings and all external factors that may influence or place demands on the person. In essence, therefore, this means the physiotherapist exerting a degree of control over:

- The physical surroundings
- Other activities within the perceivable environment
- The individual's physical position
- The person's physical and sensory interaction with both animate and inanimate aspects of the environment.

Outside direct sessions (but offering a specific impact on their conduct and outcome), it may also involve attempting to influence the client's wider ability to engage with the programme by creating the right ambient conditions, including the provision of counselling or educational programmes to effect emotional or behavioural change. As before, it also means the therapist approaching the session in a manner conducive to progress, as has been described previously.

The aspects of this approach that directly involve the physiotherapist are essentially extensions of standard physiotherapeutic practice within which, for example, various handling techniques may alter the sensory input or provide guidance for the execution of movement. Similarly, verbal instruction or feedback may be used to reinforce accurate execution or induce adaptation of a movement, or an alternative visual target, or some other form of self-monitoring may be suggested to effect more efficient motor performance.

These and many other treatment techniques influence the relationship between the individual and the environment either by inducing change via physical manipulation or altering the structure of the environment or by providing some other stimulus which in effect prompts and trains a change in performance. All that is required to enhance the productivity of therapeutic sessions in the presence of cognitive limitations is to extend the same combination of direct and indirect facilitation of the execution and practice of functional movement to those cognitive and behavioural factors that are important in the successful reacquisition of motor skills.

The guiding principle is that the combined abilities of the injured person and the structure and activity within the therapeutic environment must allow positive and progressive engagement with the chosen task. Put another way, this means that optimum performance will be achieved by case-specific tailoring of the goals, content, venue and execution of the session. To do this, the physiotherapist will need to know the deficit profile of every patient and to understand the impact of those deficits on the person's ability to deal with and engage in the rehabilitation process.

To achieve optimal engagement within a selected task, a great many factors need to be considered. For each factor that remains outside the therapist's consideration, the chances of achieving the planned session outcome will be diminished, and for each factor that is identified and dealt with appropriately there is a concomitant increase in the probability of success.

Some factors that may influence successful task engagement along with management suggestions are outlined in Tables 9.5–9.8.

It should be clear from the content of the tables that, as well as the immediate factors that may be managed within any particular session, other factors of significant impact may need to be addressed external to direct therapy sessions. Each of these factors can affect performance and success within direct therapy sessions. External factors, whether they come from non-physical deficits, the demands of other aspects of a rehabilitation programme, difficulties of adjustment, monetary pressures, relationship issues or any other source, cannot be ignored in setting realistic goals, designing treatment plans or when reappraising a programme that is failing to progress. Similarly, an acute awareness of residual factors that will continue to impact on potential future progress or the prevention of deterioration is key in estimating the likely outcome of a period of intervention or when planning service discharge and/or calculating future service needs.

Chapter 10 includes some discussion of the global service provision required to enable positive management of residual deficits and looks at the associated issues of global service provision and anticipatory service planning.

Table 9.5   Physiotherapy task engagement: impact and management of adjustment issues

Possible presenting features	Immediate management	External management	Adjustments to physical programme
Low mood or withdrawn Poor concentration Poor application	Attempt engagement on task as planned (introduction of positive activity, provision of a distracter) Communicate your observations and concerns about the person's presenting behaviour to them, if appropriate within the session Provide additional assistance to improve level of concentration	Liaise with other team members Establish any need for, and the feasibility of, providing direct help (e.g. counselling or educational support) Adjust globial intervention goals as appropriate	Suspend physical programme if unable to progress or if counterproductive Change functional focus or add additional functional goal inresponse to specific issues of concern If appropriate, include specific regime to aid venting of feelings of frustration or anger (e.g. physical workout, use of a punch bag, some form of racquet ball against a hard surface)

Table 9.6 Physiotherapy task engagement: impact and management of difficulty in sustaining attention

Possible presenting features	Immediate management	External management	Adjustments to physical programme
Boredom Apparent hearing deficit Distractibility Agitation Unable to work independently	Try to identify a point of interest (a topic or goal or an attracting stimulus within the room, such as an item of equipment) Observe factors that influence the level of sustained attention (physical or mental task, structured direction, visual, auditory or tactile factors, elapsed time) If feasible, change the environment as appropriate to the findings of the above observations	Liaise with other team members Establish limits of attention (e.g. ability to direct attention to task, factors associated with attentional loss such as fatigue or internal–external distractors) Help reduce troublesome thoughts with complementary interventions such as a recording system to support distracting memory dysfunction or counselling or educational support to reduce distress; identify and deal with troubling family or social factors	Control for identified factors within sessions, for example remove external distractors such as passing human traffic, unnecessary conversation, back-ground music; close blinds or curtains or use screens; use physical contact with precision Provide or encourage self-directed use of appropriate stimuli to re-engage attention, such as visual, auditory, verbal, tactile or movement-mediated cues Overtly link sessions with agreed functional goals and explain and reiterate the rationale to assist motivation, thus aiding internal generation of attention effort

Table 9.7 Physiotherapy task engagement: impact and management of inappropriate social behaviour

Possible presenting features	Immediate management	External management	Adjustments to physical programme
Interrupting the conversation of others Failure to appreciate inappropriate conversational content Over-familiar behaviour, failure to limit behaviour identified as unwelcome Difficulty inhibiting immediate response in demanding situations or when tired or with minimal alcohol intake	When you or others are uneasy or offended but the individual producing the behaviour is not distressed: Calmly but firmly communicate the discomfort to the offending individual, as close to the event as possible (in case of memory loss) *but* in a discrete manner When the individual is in a state of heightened arousal or there is a danger of the situation escalating: either remove the provoking factor or assist the individual to remove themselves, whichever is most feasible and *only if it is safe to do so*[a]	Liaise with other team members Agree a consistent response plus or minus a programme of intervention such as direct feedback indicating the occurrence of targeted behaviour, negotiation of contracts of behaviour, plus or minus a system of rewards, or analysis of behavioural patterns with education concerning the avoidance of provoking factors	Structure the delivery of the physical programme reflecting the agreed approach or response to the identified problems, including paying specific attention to limiting provoking factors by, for example, limiting contact between clients who are known to cause each other aggravation or avoiding unstructured time such as having to wait to commence a session Work within a contractual agreement if appropriate, being prepared to withdraw intervention if previously agreed as penalty Always seek guidance and support from colleagues experienced in the design and application of behavioural management programmes

[a]Dealing with inflamed situations is a highly skilled and always potentially dangerous activity. No professional should attempt to intervene in a situation if it increases the risk to themselves or to others, and appropriate assistance should be sought from professional security personnel or the police.

Table 9.8 Physiotherapy task engagement: impact and management of fatigue

Possible presenting features	Immediate management	External management	Adjustments to physical programme
Physical complaints such as pain, clumsiness, dizziness headache, excess sleep	Limit demands within the session	Liaise with other team members	Change the planned pace of progress, possibly working on maintenance at times rather than looking for new achievements
Cognitive complaints such as reduced concentration, increased distractibility, reduced functional performance	Exclude other sources of physical complaints	Identify influencing factors and the possibilities for introducing controls or advocating change, for example adjusting the demands of the rehabilitation programme relative to home-based demands (e.g. during school holidays), advocating a reduction in home-based demands or supporting the provision of external assistance, changing responsibilities at home to remove a particularly troublesome task, introducing additional strategies or systems as part of the global programme to improve time management and efficacy (e.g. planning and pacing activities)	Anticipate the impact of fluctuating demands at home (e.g. childcare, partner or carer illness or return to work)
Behavioural complaints such as irritability, verbal or physical outbursts, agitation or hyperactivity, sleep disturbance	Gather information and recent activity history to help ascertain whether fatigue is the issue		Anticipate the impact of new demands within the global programme (e.g. starting an educational course, period of increasing self-direction) Include education and practice regarding physical coping strategies to assist pacing (e.g. relaxation techniques, stretch regimes, short bursts of cardiovascular exercise)

Service provision

SECTION CONTENTS

10

Policy, planning and proactive management

Key Points

- Although rehabilitation can produce successful outcomes including significant positive impact on quality of life, it continues to have a low profile in both healthcare and public domains
- The development of rehabilitation as an acknowledged healthcare specialty has unfortunately coincided with a climate of extreme financial pressure in many healthcare systems, and this continues to work against service development
- There is a need for rehabilitation issues to attain equal status with other aspects of healthcare provision in the discussion of priorities and the evaluation of good practice
- Rehabilitation professionals need to be better represented on decision-making bodies and within the healthcare planning process to develop a wider appreciation of the potential social and economic impact of appropriate and timely rehabilitation
- There is a clear need for TBI rehabilitation and proactive management as evidenced by the content of this book, but the reader is reminded of the physical bias within the text and the need to look to the wider literature for a more comprehensive review of need and of effective intervention
- Models of care for TBI proposed in the literature are discussed, common themes identified and a checklist for a model service, based on a synthesis of informed opinion, is then presented

THE NATURE AND STATUS OF REHABILITATION

Rehabilitation is an important and worthwhile occupation. This feels like a vital statement to make and, while it may seem obvious in the context of this book, it is not automatically regarded as either in the financially and professionally competitive world of healthcare provision. Furthermore, in the wider world beyond healthcare provision, rehabilitation is, in general, poorly understood. In terms of investment – and of media interest – it continues to be overshadowed by the more glamorous, more miraculous, aspects of healthcare practice.

Rehabilitation is not a dramatic, headline-grabbing activity, it is rarely hi-tech and its effects are infrequently instantaneous. When there is positive effect, it may not be easily appreciated by the uninformed outside observer and it may take a series of stepwise progressions over a period of time to produce a clearly recognizable impact on an individual's life in terms of functional change.

Sometimes intervention is not even targeted at achieving positive change but at preventing, slowing or managing deterioration, and this makes the assessment or observation of efficacy doubly difficult. Positive treatment effects may be perceived only by the recipient, who may appreciate the arrested deterioration, or by those close to them, who may observe improved quality of life or find their caring role reduced or easier to execute. Therefore, although rehabilitation professionals, recipients and their carers know that given time and appropriate intervention rehabilitation can produce significant positive impact on quality of life, it continues to have a low profile in both the healthcare and public domains.

COMPETING FACTORS AND EXTERNAL INFLUENCES

Rehabilitation has a relatively short history compared with more traditional areas of medical practice, developing mainly over the second half of the twentieth century. It is unfortunate that recent progress in the development of rehabilitation as an acknowledged healthcare specialty has coincided with substantial pressures on the funding of health and social care throughout the industrialized nations. And, as the possibilities for life preservation continue to increase, often with associated increased financial demands, it is hard to stem the flow of resources within finite, pressurized, budgets towards established acute care and away from developing restorative services.

Furthermore, in recent times, when acute care has come under financial pressure, one of the main money-saving strategies has been to reduce the number of bed-days and often consequently to squeeze the period of associated access to concurrent rehabilitation.

In the UK, there have been particular problems related to the speed of implementation of these so-called efficiency changes, to their unplanned nature and their frequent enactment with apparent lack of awareness of the impact on non-medical services. These changes have also taken place within a competitive business environment (relatively foreign to UK practitioners) brought about by the establishment of National Health Service (NHS) Trusts with their business-led approach to driving down the cost of healthcare.

The service ethos, which previously would have been more concerned with the longitudinal outcome for individual patients, was forced to change to a focus on increasing the number of patients seen and/or producing the same outcomes over a shorter period of contact. The majority of the measures employed to assess these efficiency improvements have been based on a purely medical model of medical consultant waiting times, hospital admission and discharge numbers, and numbers of surgical operations. At best this has had no direct link with rehabilitation provision, and at worst is has produced demands to process more people through the system.

During this time of rapid change, many rehabilitation professionals have consistently found themselves in a reactive stance, running to catch up, and expending more energy managing change than developing practice. Many have also experienced a sense of powerlessness in not being able fully to exercise their professional judgement in relation to intervention approaches, speed of progression and readiness for discharge because of the sheer pressure of achieving speedy discharge, based on the medical analysis of appropriate discharge status and the increasingly pervasive argument that people, in general, are better off in their own home. All in all, the squeeze on acute care budgets has resulted in increased limitations on the delivery of rehabilitation within acute care provision without this necessarily being acknowledged, without a clear analysis of its impact, and without planned provision of alternative services.

It has been possible in some instances to respond positively to such changes in patterns of healthcare delivery and to achieve continued high standards of rehabilitation or even improve models of care by implementing changes in the practice and delivery of rehabilitation services via outreach or outpatient provision. However, this positive picture does not apply to all enforced changes, and effective restructuring has proved possible only in relation to the management of certain pathologies or concerning follow-up after some surgical procedures, and where local circumstances have allowed a speedy reorganization of service delivery.

Where local circumstances have not allowed a dynamic response, or when it has been inappropriate or financially impossible to provide suitable alternative community-based provision, the outcome for those requiring rehabilitation has been a diminished service. Some aspects of rehabilitation have been negatively affected simply by virtue of the fact that they happened to develop alongside acute-care provision and, since the rehabilitation aspect of the service has been regarded as peripheral to the core business of medical and nursing care, it has been sacrificed.

The growing assumption that all rehabilitation services are better delivered at home or in the local area has been a powerful factor in promoting or excusing some changes, but this is simply an assumption and the truth is that in the vast majority of cases comparative studies of efficacy or cost have not even been attempted. It may not have been essential or even appropriate for all hospital-based rehabilitation services to continue to be provided as part of acute provision, but some aspects of rehabilitation and/or periods of management within a process of rehabilitation are more effectively and efficiently delivered from a residential base.

The problem has been, and continues to be, one of getting discussion of these basic issues on to the planning agenda and ensuring an objective and informed decision-making process. This is the environment within which attempts to develop rehabilitation for TBI survivors have taken place over recent years in the UK.

CHANGING POLICIES AND CHANGING EMPHASIS

Fortunately, it would seem that it is now accepted beyond staffing groups within the NHS that the simple application of business management models and free market principles will not achieve the anticipated financial containment. A change in government has brought about a change in emphasis and it is increasingly accepted that, as well as adopting sensible business practice where applicable, healthcare providers, in order to contain the spiralling cost of healthcare, must also examine what they currently do and, if appropriate, be prepared to change their practice.

However, as the purely business approach was not the complete answer to the problem of limited resources, neither will be the process of basing practice on best evidence. Within a finite budget, priorities will always need to be identified and in the delivery of a national service, like the NHS, within a democracy, priorities and exclusions need to reflect the opinions of society in general.

DEFINING PRIORITIES IN HEALTHCARE PROVISION

In the UK, the whole debate concerning priorities in healthcare provision and the need to equate service delivery with the available resources has now begun to enter a more public forum. Here, as elsewhere in the developed world, both government and the general public are trying to reconcile the previously accepted principle of universal access to basic health and social care, seen as a marker of a civilized society, with the current less than universal willingness of taxpayers to make sufficient financial contribution to fund all the services required to meet this worthy aim.

The public debate is as yet selective, disjointed, and often based around emotive issues. There is still a long way to go before there is wide recognition that, even with the most efficiently delivered services, the impact of having finite resources is that choices have to be made. While this remains the case, the low public profile and limited emotive impact of rehabilitation provision will continue to work against galvanizing wider support for the development of rehabilitation services. There is, therefore, a need to develop a wider appreciation of the potential social and economic impact of appropriate and timely rehabilitation.

QUALITY AND EFFECTIVE PRACTICE

Action on determining priorities within the health industry itself (via the process of defining effective practice) is being pushed forward by the new central approach heralded by governmental change. The strategy to modernize healthcare provision in the UK is now being described in terms of a national quality framework (Department of Health 1998), with the stated intent of having a national service framework with clear service standards.

These national standards and more clinically specific guidelines will be developed and communicated via the National Institute for Clinical Excellence, which is intended to raise the standard and speed of information to be disseminated, and to help ensure wider and more even distribution of available information. Easy access to this and other local, national and international evidence sources will be supported by developing Internet connections, intranet facilities and other data management systems. The effective application of disseminated knowledge and the incorporation of guidelines into practice will also be formally monitored.

As a result of new legislation, each subunit of the NHS now has a statutory duty to deliver on clinical standards as well as financial targets, and organizational structures are being adapted to recognize the demands of this new dimension, known as clinical governance. All these developments have added impetus to the quality and priority debate within healthcare provision.

Each professional body has in turn embraced the ideal of practice based on best evidence to ensure a high standard of care but there will need to be significant cultural change before we see meaningful savings as a result of the discontinuation of ineffective and inefficient practice. In addition, there is the danger that those professions and clinical areas that have an established body of knowledge from which detailed guidelines may more easily be derived will again have advantage over newer or less academically mature sectors, like rehabilitation.

There is, therefore, an ongoing need for rehabilitation issues to attain equal status with other aspects of healthcare provision in the development, synthesis and application of good evidence to everyday practice and within the planning process.

COLLABORATIVE PLANNING

The changes in central policy, as well as aiming for quality through the application of evidence, are also promoting a more collaborative approach to service planning and provision, supporting the merger of Trusts and the development of associate hospital groupings. Similarly, local community-based service needs are to be determined via primary care groups, managed by committees comprising, in the main, local healthcare professionals. It would seem, therefore, that a number of structures and forums are being established in the UK to facilitate knowledge-based developments and inclusive debate to help planners and practitioners to make good choices concerning service delivery within the confines of whatever resources are available at any particular time.

However, to date, the membership or proposed composition of the new influential organizations remains heavily biased towards the medical and nursing professions, which does not seem to be the best way of ensuring inclusive debate or of accessing the wide range of knowledge, expertise and alternative perspectives that are held in the wider healthcare community.

It is therefore unclear how informed the internal healthcare debate will be and whether, for example, the potential for therapeutic intervention to reduce dependency, and therefore cost, will be fully appreciated. It is also unclear how rehabilitation professionals will be able to influence the cultural change required to ensure the necessary redistribution of funds within the system to support goal-directed rehabilitation, adjustment and planned management programmes.

The apparent lack of progress in central recognition of the value of rehabilitation, and of the potential of rehabilitation professionals to inform the global health and social care debate, would seem to indicate that there is still a great deal of education and promotional work to be done clearly to set out rehabilitation as a regulated, purposeful, activity that empowers the individual to take control and responsibility, and that it is not a soft, paternalistic, caring, activity that induces a dependency culture.

We have somehow to move beyond the planning and management culture that sees consultation with doctors as essential, that will often consult nurses, and that sometimes remembers to inform other professionals, to a culture with wider and more flexible discussion forums, where representation is defined by the nature of the task in hand. This proposed cultural change should not be seen as an attack on the clinical expertise of nurses or doctors, or in any way as an attempt to devalue the crucial role of both professions within the healthcare system. It does reflect a demand to end an effective veto on alternative viewpoints or strategic approaches that results from the failure of decision-making bodies to reflect the true multiprofessional nature of service provision.

Similarly, the analysis, evaluation and planning of rehabilitation services, especially in the case of complex provision such as for the TBI population, also need to reflect the multiagency nature of effective provision and be informed by the experience of TBI survivors and those who have shared the experience with them. Thus, service analysis and planning should be derived from information gathered from a full range of statutory and voluntary agencies, from a range of professions, from the published literature and from local knowledge of real outcomes. In this way decisions will be made from a background of detailed understanding, incorporating an appropriately wide perspective and, when the question of investment arises, the analysis will then reflect the cost of service provision as a whole and the full benefits to society rather than only purely local factors.

Widening the ethical and economic debate

Just as collaborative planning can have the effect of widening the scope of economic analysis, the decision-making process is also likely to highlight moral and ethical issues. A further effect would be to raise the profile and understanding of the value of rehabilitation across professions and agencies by raising awareness of the real longitudinal impact of disability and also by illustrating the positive results of effective intervention or management.

Involvement of rehabilitation professionals in collaborative planning and similar multiprofessional forums will contribute to the process of establishing rehabilitation on an equal footing within the health agenda. It will also move forward the professional healthcare priorities debate so that it widens beyond issues such as the best value for money drug, the most effective form of surgical intervention or what duties can be passed from doctor to nurse.

There are many issues concerning approach to intervention, of basic principles of service delivery, and of priorities for investment that have yet to be debated openly. In relation to TBI services there are a number of wider issues requiring attention, for example the discussion of opportunities for injury prevention and health promotion, proactive disability management and, of particular importance, the issue of responsibility for longitudinal health and social care. From both an ethical and an economic standpoint, there needs to be open debate of the long-term responsibilities that emanate from our compulsion to intervene to save life.

At present it appears that the practice of making every effort to save life at the time of injury is accepted and not open to discussion. Equally, the need for surgical intervention, intensive care support and for hospital care until medically stable is not questioned.

In contrast, although advanced skills and knowledge for saving lives have been developed, survival rates have rocketed and the severity of residual deficits has been reduced, rehabilitation services are often not available, not adequate, or not accepted as being necessary. This observation is made all the more poignant by the relatively high cost of acute and subacute care, which is seen as mandatory, in contrast to the low-tech post-acute provision to guide and support the transition into, and stability within, the real world.

The principles and values that underpin the automatic practice of intervening to save life must be applied equally to reintegration back into the community. It is simply not ethical to stabilize an injured person's medical condition because medical knowledge allows us to do so and then restrict access to rehabilitation knowledge either through failure to recognize the need or the potential benefit to the individual. It is equally unsatisfactory to limit service provision because of financial constraints within the health sector without consideration of the longer-term cost, for example in terms of other social provision, other health services, the criminal justice system or in diminished income in terms of tax receipts.

INFORMING SERVICE PLANNING

What knowledge and information can we, then, contribute to the service development process for TBI?

Facts and opinions contained in this book

The incidence, pathophysiology and potential effects of TBI are described in the early sections of this book, indicating the size and scope of the problem. Subsequently, a whole range of observable deficits, their direct functional effect and their wider personal and social impact have also been presented and discussed along with suggestions for intervention and management, including suggestions for the effective organization of interdisciplinary teamwork.

However, while this text emphasizes the interactive nature of deficits, the importance of specialized global assessment, and teamwork, it has by necessity a bias towards the factors that directly concern physical therapy or have an influence on its practice. Although the information presented does strongly support the need for multiprofessional and multiagency provision for those recovering from TBI, it is not a comprehensive rehabilitation text. It should be noted, for example, that there is more research evidence to support the effects of intervention aimed at non-physical deficits that is not referred to in this text because of its physical focus, but that would be essential to consider when reviewing evidence for efficacy within the rehabilitation process.

None the less, it should be clear from the foregoing chapters that the residual effects of TBI are to some degree lifelong in many cases and that their impact may be felt beyond the individual, often within the immediate family and sometimes significantly more widely. It should also be apparent that if the potential complexity of the effects of even some mild or moderate injuries is acknowledged, and the knowledge and skills possessed by a number of crucial disciplines are combined to address the complex outcome within a single service, then rehabilitation, adjustment and reintegration become a distinct prospect for the great majority of individuals following TBI.

It is accepted that detailed proof of efficacy is not yet available because of the relative youth of the discipline, the scarcity of multiprofessional provision and the limited investment in in-depth research. Lack of documented proof of positive effect does not necessarily mean, however, that the positive effect is not there, and throughout this book I have tried to illustrate via real case examples the positive outcome for patients and their families of a thoughtful, collaborative approach to service provision. I have also argued that therapists involved in planned collaborative provision, rather than in isolated single-discipline services, experience a higher level of professional satisfaction, which in turn produces a positive effect on the service in terms of stability and the development of advanced knowledge and therapeutic skills.

A wider perspective from the published literature

Like many rehabilitation professionals, my expertise in relation to strategic planning on a population basis is limited and I do not write from an in-depth knowledge of theoretical models, activity-based formulae or any other form of academic analysis. What we do know about is what happens when services are not adequate or appropriately integrated, where the system fails, and what practical solutions may be appropriate.

In addition, our knowledge of the population and observation of their needs, combined with the problem-solving skills we use in everyday clinical practice, offer a potentially rich resource that can assist planners and policymakers in reaching informed decisions. Indeed, while hard research data and cost–benefit analyses are not yet available for many service models or specific interventions, a number of experienced clinicians have described an overview of service needs or proposed service models in the literature. Some of these are discussed below.

This approach does not reflect an attitude that fails to accept the need for definitive research; indeed, several of the authors of these papers and chapters have been and continue to be active in robust research activity. It is more of a pragmatic response to a hugely complex issue, which cannot simply wait for definitive experimental proof of efficacy, and where in fact efficacy cannot be assessed until provision is established. Where available, research evidence has been included in each of these analyses, but in the main these publications represent an interpretative synthesis of evidence, knowledge and experience, producing informed opinion.

In 1985, an editorial review of presentations given at the Medical Disability Society's symposium on better services for head injury appeared in the *British Medical Journal* (Gloag 1985) which, in effect, outlined both the positive and negative aspects of UK services at the time. One negative aspect described was that of inappropriately placed TBI survivors still resident in acute hospital beds years after injury.

These individuals were assessed as having rehabilitation potential but had no accessible rehabilitation placement. Another cause for concern, with regard to a group of patients who *did* receive early inpatient rehabilitation, was the finding that despite the progress achieved during the hospital stay many became inactive and increasingly distressed after hospital discharge. It was noted in particular that help was not available at the point when individuals had begun to realize that a full return to their previous lifestyle was not to be.

In contrast, another study that was quoted reported positive outcomes measured 5 years' postinjury, including successful return to work. However, it was also made clear that support for subjects within this group had been given over years rather than months.

In light of the variance in interventions and outcomes, another presentation proposed that a coherent network of services should be set up to ensure equality of access and to prevent individuals missing out on the help they needed and would benefit from. It was recognized that, to achieve such an extended network of services and to develop better forms of intervention, there was a need for education across a wide spectrum of professions and that clinical staff also needed to develop additional skills. Equally important for the success and future development of the proposed service network was the need to include a research mechanism within the service model, in order to evaluate progress and to build knowledge systematically.

The service model outlined in the 1985 report was described in more detail in 1989 by Eames and Wood (1989), a neuropsychiatrist and a neuropsychologist with significant experience in TBI rehabilitation and management in the UK and the USA. As well as the service principles previously outlined, this expanded version included a description of seven different subpopulations, differentiated by their patterns of recovery and by different service needs. Detailed suggestions as to what type of service, if any, would be most effective in meeting the needs of each particular group were also made.

Eames and Wood's service recommendations ranged from the provision of advice (sometimes treatment) and careful follow-up for those at the mild end of the spectrum, through comprehensive and intensive rehabilitation programmes delivered by services with special TBI expertise for those with slow to resolve deficits, to the need for those with dominant behavioural disorders to have rehabilitation programmes that addressed both the behavioural disorder and other residual deficits in tandem.

One of the specific subpopulations highlighted by Eames and Wood, which is of continuing relevance to physical rehabilitation, concerns those who experience a very long coma and have very severe physical deficits, but who continue to benefit from rehabilitation for a very long time (years), and who often have an initial latent period before their positive response to intervention becomes apparent. They also recognized, and clearly describe, the special service needs of those who remain in a persistent vegetative state, and the needs of their families.

Eames and Wood, within their defined populations, make a clear distinction between those with behavioural disorders that respond to behavioural management programmes and those that do not, highlighting the latter as a group with distinct management needs. They assert that people who experience severe non-traumatic insults to the brain (hypoxia, ischaemia or hypoglycaemia), and who may or may not have also sustained a TBI, often present serious management challenges in the form of behavioural disorders that are apparently resistant to behavioural modification techniques. While they clearly state that this group's adverse reaction to behavioural modification programmes necessitates that they be treated differently, they are equally straightforward in their admission that no alternative satisfactory treatment solution has yet been found.

As well as outlining the necessary component parts of a comprehensive service, Eames and Wood consider other factors in the design of a successful rehabilitation service. Within the discussion of these influencing factors is a strong message of the need for the physical structure, ambience and staff attitude within the service *not* to reflect an illness–caring relationship. Rather, there should be an ethos that suggests a positive, constructive progression towards the real world, with a strong sense of belief in the possible and collaborative working relationships between all concerned, including an appropriate spread of responsibility.

They consider recovery and rehabilitation to cover four overlapping periods: acute, intermediate, resettlement and long-term, and outline some of the required service content for each stage. In the case of long-term support, they make three specific observations. The first is that the numbers involved will be lessened by more effective and efficient early rehabilitation efforts. Second, they make the point that, for some injured people, long term means for the rest of their lives. Third, they suggest that for some others the knowledge that support is potentially there, if required, is enough to ensure their continued success.

In summary, Eames and Wood (1989, p. 45) argue for: 'coherent organization which takes account of the whole range of injuries, and seeks to identify and follow victims until they have re-established themselves in as satisfactory a social niche as possible'. They also see as essential that the service is dedicated to TBI, that rehabilitation teams are interdisciplinary in nature, have close links with acute teams and community services, accumulate expertise, undertake research, and evaluate and develop their professional roles in line with the needs of the TBI population. This professional development might include developing skills outside normal professional experience and learning to appreciate the potential of other fields to contribute to the process of rehabilitation.

It is ironic that, at the time this detailed analysis of service needs was being written, a survey of facilities for adult TBI rehabilitation in the UK was published (Cockburn and Gatherer 1988), with the main conclusion that 'specific provision, tailored to the rehabilitation needs of adults after head injury appear[ed] to be rare.' This paper also highlighted that the geographical distribution of services that did exist was skewed towards the south of England, indicating that large parts of the country were without any specialized service.

However, this lack of service provision was not limited to the UK. In Australia, Burke (1987), from a distinguished background in wider rehabilitation and recent experience in a new venture of specialized TBI rehabilitation, was moved to outline the need for a planned system of care for TBI survivors based on the same comprehensive level of service afforded to those with spinal cord injuries. While there are some differences in the descriptive language, with aspects of the proposed service appearing under different headings or labels, there is a striking similarity in the overall picture of the proposed service.

Like Eames and Wood, Burke identifies four primary service components: specialized acute trauma care, acute rehabilitation, outpatient rehabilitation and community support. He also describes the need for a continuum of care for each individual patient within a planned, flexible system, and recognizes the need for special considerations for subpopulations: 'slow stream rehabilitation' for the group that responds slowly to initial intervention, 'psychiatric rehabilitation' for those with predominantly behavioural disorders and 'vocational rehabilitation' for those who have potential to return to the workplace, but who need specialist assistance to get there.

Burke's system is presented as an interlinking cycle of care; again, like Eames and Wood, he stresses the need for overlap and the facility to move into any aspect of provision at the time when it is appropriate to the needs of the individual. Burke clearly identifies the key role of assessment services 'to enable highly qualified assessment of individual needs to be made from time to time'. This includes specialist assessment as part of community-based follow-up services that should 'support patients and their families for life, and direct individuals to expert assessment services as required' Burke (1987, p. 197).

Oddy and colleagues (1989) also proposed a model service encompassing several subcomponents through which individuals should progress as related to their needs. Consistent with the recommendations of the previously cited authors, both residential and non-residential rehabilitation programmes are advocated, along with provision to deal with behavioural problems, vocational issues and supported living, including services to meet the needs of both the injured person and their families and carers.

In discussing issues of provision, they suggest that it is not essential for each component part of the service to be managed by the same agency and that there may indeed be advantages to be gained from cross-agency provision. They do stress, however, that clear channels of communication and effective coordination are essential across the service as a whole, however it is organized. They also acknowledge that the delivery of such a comprehensive service (in the UK) would require an increased number of rehabilitation professionals and improved methods of education and training for all professions to develop the appropriate knowledge and skill to deliver an appropriately specialized service.

All three analyses produced by Eames and Wood, Burke, and Oddy et al highlight that the efficacy of any TBI service is dependent on timely service provided by skilled practitioners and, while all three proposals suggest that further developments and service evaluations should be based on formal research, equally they warn against failing to evaluate the results of a whole service or of evaluating services provided by inexperienced practitioners.

Greenwood and McMillan, in the first of two linked papers, reviewed current UK provision, assessed its status with reference to available research evidence and advanced a series of principles of good practice as a basis for service organization and development (Greenwood and McMillan 1993). In the second paper they applied the principles to a logical service progression, giving more details at each stage (McMillan and Greenwood 1993).

Their review highlighted that, at the beginning of the last decade of the twentieth century, there was still 'virtually no specialist rehabilitation and retraining to return the individual to an independent and productive role in society, (p. 250) and that there was continuing evidence of inappropriately placed individuals and of people being discharged to the care of relatives without management advice, support or follow-up. There was no logical progression through services that did exist, hurdles between cross-agency provision and, although a few specialized brain injury units were identified both in the public and independent sectors, the total numbers provided for remained small.

Taking into account the available evidence on efficacy of interventions and the characteristics of the TBI population, Greenwood and McMillan argued that ideally service provision should be specialist and categorical, in the same way that it is for spinal injury, and that rehabilitation should start as early as possible and consist of a menu of services to cater for the different stages of recovery after injury. They also stressed the need for timely access to the appropriate aspect of service and the need for many elements of provision to be sited somewhere other than in a hospital setting to emphasize the move towards independence and the educational and training nature of the service. They emphasized the need for integrated teamwork, for the communal setting and review of a series of functional goals, and for individual discipline skills to be used within a wider cognitive–behavioural context. Finally, in terms of basic principles, they described the need for service provision for family members in their own right.

The second of the two linked papers included a clear description of the operational components of a model service and discussed some of the organizational issues and important factors governing the appropriate approach for each component (McMillan and Greenwood 1993). The service model recommended is based on an early transition from the medical model of care to that which is neurobehavioural and educational in nature. Crucially, while each component or service module is seen to be distinct, it is also *integrated* into the overall service and *provided at a time that is appropriate to the changing demands of the patient*. Equally important is the proactive nature of the service design, anticipating the potential deficits and complications whether physical, behavioural or social, and intervening to minimize their development.

McMillan and Greenwood concluded that there is a need for a variety of residential and outpatient service components, as detailed in Box 10.1. These components address in some detail the same set of progressions identified by the three previously reviewed authors, from acute medical care, through acute rehabilitation, integrative rehabilitation and episodic review. Again, the need for flexibility in the system is stressed to allow access to vital components at the appropriate time and the design of the provision takes into account the lifelong needs of a number of TBI survivors.

McMillan and Greenwood also raised the issue of professional training and skill development needs, and suggested strongly that professional bodies should facilitate the development of accredited courses and that staff from specialist centres should advise and educate other professionals. They are also clear that, while the basic service outline and some of the recommended content could be defended in the light of

---

Box 10.1 Operational classification of modules providing residential and outpatient acute, late and long-term rehabilitation for severely brain-injured adults (McMillan and Greenwood 1993)

Residential

1. Acute (until 9–12 months postinjury)
   a. In surgical ward
   b. 'Brain injury' units
2. Coma management and persistent vegetative state
3. Late (from 6 months to years postinjury)
   a. Extended acute ('physical') rehabilitation
   b. Transitional living and vocational programmes
   c. Behavioural units
4. Long-term (after 12–24 months postinjury)[a]
   a. Family or own home + carer and respite
   b. Supervised group home or hostel
   c. Categorical provision for
      (i) Severe physical disablement
      (ii) Severe cognitive impairment

Outpatient

1. Any interval postinjury
   a. Episodic access to medical and other professions
   b. Day programmes for training in:
      (i) Independent living skills
      (ii) Emotional and social skills
      (iii) Vocational and educational re-entry

[a] In conjunction with day centre, recreational, educational provision and sheltered or supported work.

---

current knowledge, there is also a pressing need for local evaluation and longitudinal research.

Recurring themes

There appears to be a broad consensus regarding the global picture of need for rehabilitation, adjustment and management services for the adult TBI population across the four opinions reviewed. There is also broad agreement in terms of the necessary components, the need for organizational integration, interdisciplinary teamwork, professionals with advanced knowledge and skills, and a systematic programme of service evaluation and innovative research.

These conclusions and those drawn from the content of this book are further validated by the recommendations generated more recently in the USA from the National Institutes of Health Consensus Development Conference (NIH Consensus Statement 1998), which state:

- Rehabilitation services should be matched to the needs, strengths, and capacities of each person with TBI and modified as those needs change over time
- Rehabilitation programs for persons with moderate or severe TBI should be interdisciplinary and comprehensive

- Rehabilitation of persons with TBI should include cognitive and behavioral assessment and intervention
- Persons with TBI and their families should have the opportunity to play an integral role in the planning and design of their individualized rehabilitation programs and associated research endeavors
- Persons with TBI should have access to rehabilitative services through the entire course of recovery, which may last for many years after injury
- Substance abuse evaluation and treatment should be a component of rehabilitation treatment programs
- Medications used for behavioral management have significant side effects in persons with TBI, can impede rehabilitation progress, and should therefore only be used in compelling circumstances
- Medications used for cognitive enhancement can be effective, but benefits should be carefully evaluated and documented in each individual
- Community-based, nonmedical services should be components of the extended care and rehabilitation available to people with TBI. These include, but are not necessarily limited to, clubhouses for socialization; day programs and social skill development programs; supported living programs and independent living centers; supported employment programs, formal education programs at all levels; case manager programs to support practical life skill redevelopment and to help navigate through the public assistance and medical–rehabilitative care systems; and consumer, peer support programs
- Families and significant others provide support for many people with TBI. To do so effectively, they themselves should receive support. This can include in-home assistance from home health aides or personal care attendants, daytime and overnight respite care, and ongoing counselling
- Rehabilitation efforts should include modification of the individual's home, social, and work environments to enable fuller participation in all venues
- Specialized programs are needed to identify and treat persons with mild TBI
- Specialized, interdisciplinary, and comprehensive treatment programs are necessary to address the particular medical, rehabilitation, social, family, and educational needs of young and school age children with TBI
- Specialized, interdisciplinary, and comprehensive treatment programs are necessary to address the particular medical, rehabilitation, social, family, and educational needs of persons older than age 65 with TBI
- Educational programs are needed to increase the degree to which community care providers are aware of the problems experienced by persons with TBI.

Furthermore, the consensus statement details 30 specific areas of immediate research need, many of which relate to developing and evaluating interventions.

There is, without doubt, a global recognition by TBI practitioners of the type and extent of the needs of this population, general agreement regarding the scope of support required, and acceptance of the need to develop knowledge and test practice via the research process. However, in practice there remain significant financial, organizational and logistical barriers to achieving the multiprofessional, multiagency cooperation necessary to achieve even a basic level of service integration and to ensure smooth and appropriate progression through that service.

CARE PATHWAYS, MANAGING TRANSITIONS AND THE EFFECTIVE USE OF RESOURCES

A straightforward approach to beginning the process of integration, which is gaining support in many health and social care settings, is that of the defined care pathway. Central to this approach is:

- The identification of existing components of service
- Negotiation and agreement of the extent and limits of responsibility for each service component, including inclusion and exclusion criteria, expected outcomes, standard timescales or other limiting factors
- Negotiation and agreement between services of the preferred pathway of care to be followed by the service recipient
- Agreed mechanisms for movement between service components
- Procedures for resolution of disputes between service components and procedures for regular review.

While, in theory, this would appear to be a suitable mechanism for ensuring appropriate movement of individuals through a TBI service, the variety of subpopulations and their differing needs makes this a fairly complex process.

For example, a working party that I was involved with identified five primary categories at service entry with differing medical needs and six community-based categories requiring a range of service intensities and with the potential for people from almost all acute categories to progress through a variety of service pathways and eventually map on to almost any of the community categories.

As identified by Burke (1987), decisions regarding onward referral were seen to be dependent upon a combination of expert assessment leading to knowledge of the potential of the individual and full awareness of the scope of service provision available from each service. While it was agreed that care pathways would guide and assist this process by describing the possibilities and relevant actions, the decision culminating in accurate and timely onward referral was still regarded as a highly skilled one. Similarly, the decision to accept a referral and the detailed programme plan within each service component should also be based on an understanding of global need and a full awareness of the potential contribution from other service components.

Therefore, even if clear pathways are developed for all the main scenarios, movement through the service will always be complex and potentially confusing for those who have to do so. In this regard we must also take into account the issues of awareness and adjustment highlighted in earlier chapters and appreciate that, even with care pathways in place, the person with TBI, and possibly more importantly their immediate carers, will need guidance to understand what constitutes the correct service and to understand its significance. They may also require assistance to communicate effectively with those delivering the service.

In practice, I have experience of both these functions of carer–family support and service identification and facilitation of appropriate referral being effectively managed by a small team of specialist TBI social workers (Herbert et al 1995).

The organization of TBI provision over a set geographical area needs more than the simple care pathway approach for reasons other than those already outlined. For example, not all provision can be provided locally, and individuals may at times have to access specialist service components away from their local area. To keep track of these people and other groups, for example those on review, appropriate data management systems and review procedures need to be employed. Furthermore, I would argue that, given the complexities already outlined, the need for multiprofessional and cross-agency collaboration, planning, review and financial risk sharing, there should be an easily convenable cross-agency forum, with a designated chair and/or someone with the stated responsibility for ensuring that an efficient integrated service becomes and remains a reality.

CHECKLIST FOR A MODEL SERVICE

PRINCIPLES AND APPROACH

- Interdisciplinary, cross-agency working
- Early transition to cognitive–behavioural model
- Positive and forward looking
- Collaborative, with survivors and families
- Flexible system, timely access
- Continuum of care
- Intervention and progression based on expert assessment
- Life-long support or access to reassessment, where applicable

SERVICE COMPONENTS

- Skilled, efficient paramedical service
- Knowledgeable, skilled hospital emergency service
- Easy access to skilled neurosurgical advice and intervention
- Acute or subacute residential interdisciplinary rehabilitation service
- Direct support, education and guidance for families from acute to community
- Access to provision for dominant behavioural disorders
- Access to provision for the slow to respond
- Access to provision for those in a persistent vegetative state

- Non-residential interdisciplinary rehabilitation service
- Access to specialist vocational training
- Community-based assessment and review service, including provision for slow to resolve mild injuries
- Community-based long-term management service for those with persistent severe deficits, including skilled care and a variety of options for supported living
- Respite care

ORGANIZATIONAL AND SUPPORTING FACTORS

- Data management system
- Care pathways
- Cross-agency planning and monitoring group
- Named person with organizational overview, authority and responsibility
- High level of postgraduate education
- Collaborative research and evaluation
- Effective education and support for non-professional staff

REFERENCES

Burke D 1987 Planning a system of care for head injuries. Brain Injury 1(2):189–198
Cockburn J, Gatherer A 1988 Facilities for rehabilitation of adults after head injury. Clinical Rehabilitation 2:315–318
Department of Health 1998 A first class service: quality in the new NHS. NHS Executive, Wetherby, UK
Eames P, Wood R 1989 The structure and content of a head injury rehabilitation service. In: Wood R L, Eames P (eds) Models of brain injury rehabilitation, 1st edn. Chapman & Hall, London, p 31
Gloag D 1985 Services for people after head injury. British Medical Journal 291:557–558
Greenwood R, McMillan T M 1993 Models of rehabilitation programmes for the brain-injured adult. I: Current provision, efficacy and good practice. Clinical Rehabilitation 7:248–255
Herbert C, Garber J, Parker J S 1995 Family focus – model of service to traumatic brain injury families. Second European Neurorehabilitation conference, September 1995, University of Leeds, Leeds, UK
McMillan T, Greenwood R 1993 Models of rehabilitation programmes for the brain-injured adult. II: Model services and suggestions for change in the UK. Clinical Rehabilitation 7:346–355
NIH Consensus Statement 1998 Rehabilitation of persons with traumatic brain injury. NIH Consensus Statement Online 16(1):1–41
Oddy M, Bonham E, McMillan T M, Stroud A, Rickard S 1989 A comprehensive service for the rehabilitation and long-term care of head injury survivors. Clinical Rehabilitation 3:253–259

Index

Note: page numbers in **bold** refer to figures. The abbreviation TBI stands for traumatic brain injury.